NCLEX-1

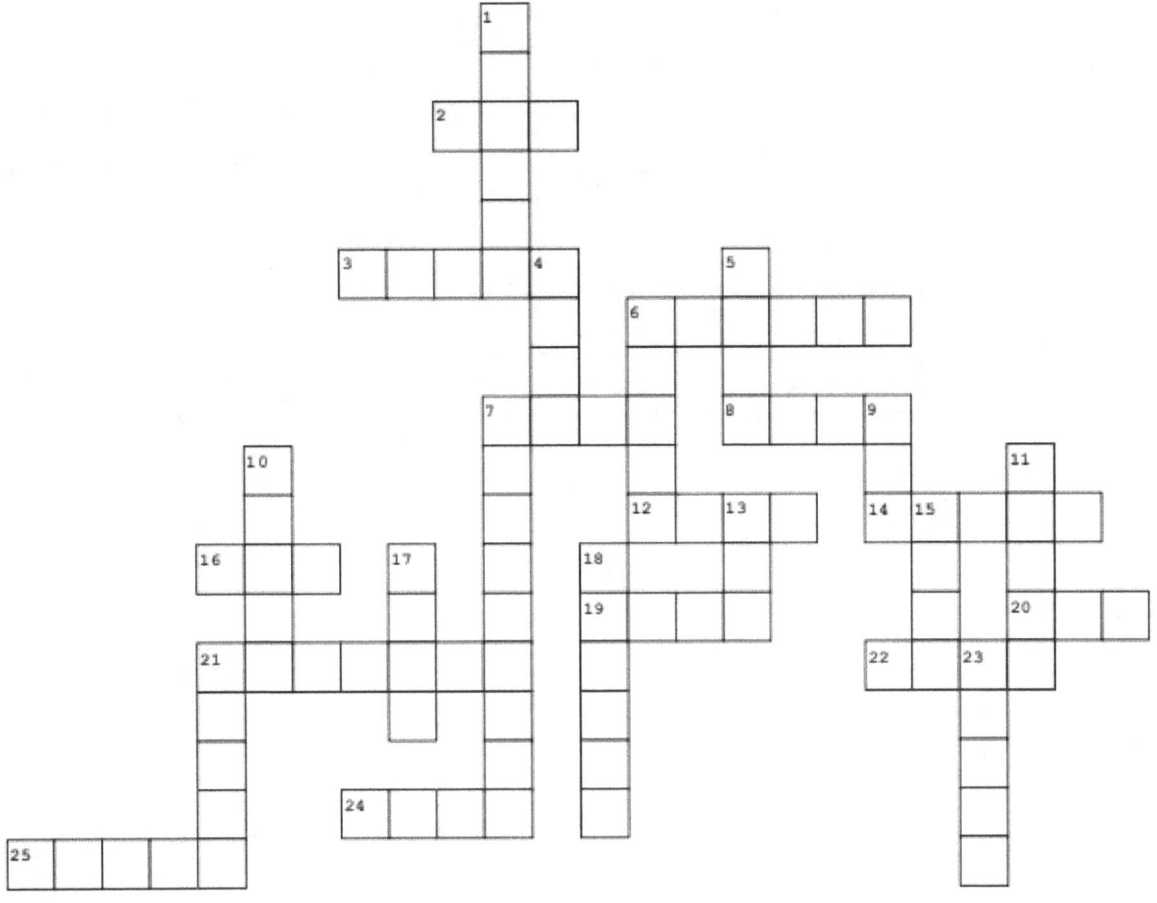

Across
2. medical meaning for brach
3. medical meaning for sphygm
6. medical terminology for remove
7. medical meaning for oste
8. medical meaning for derm
12. medical terminology for gland
14. medical terminology for hardening

Down
1. medical meaning for trans
4. medical terminology for inside
5. medical terminology for inflammation
6. medical terminology for swelling
7. medical meaning for spir
9. medical terminology for nose

16. medical meaning for eryth
19. medical terminology for below
20. medical meaning for cost
21. medical meaning for gastro
22. medical terminology for tooth
24. medical meaning for pneumon
25. medical terminology for above

10. medical meaning for steth
11. medical meaning for cardi
13. medical terminology for outside
15. medical terminology for cell
17. medical terminology for dark blue
18. medical terminology for blood cloth
21. medical meaning for glyc
23. medical meaning for neur

NCLEX-2

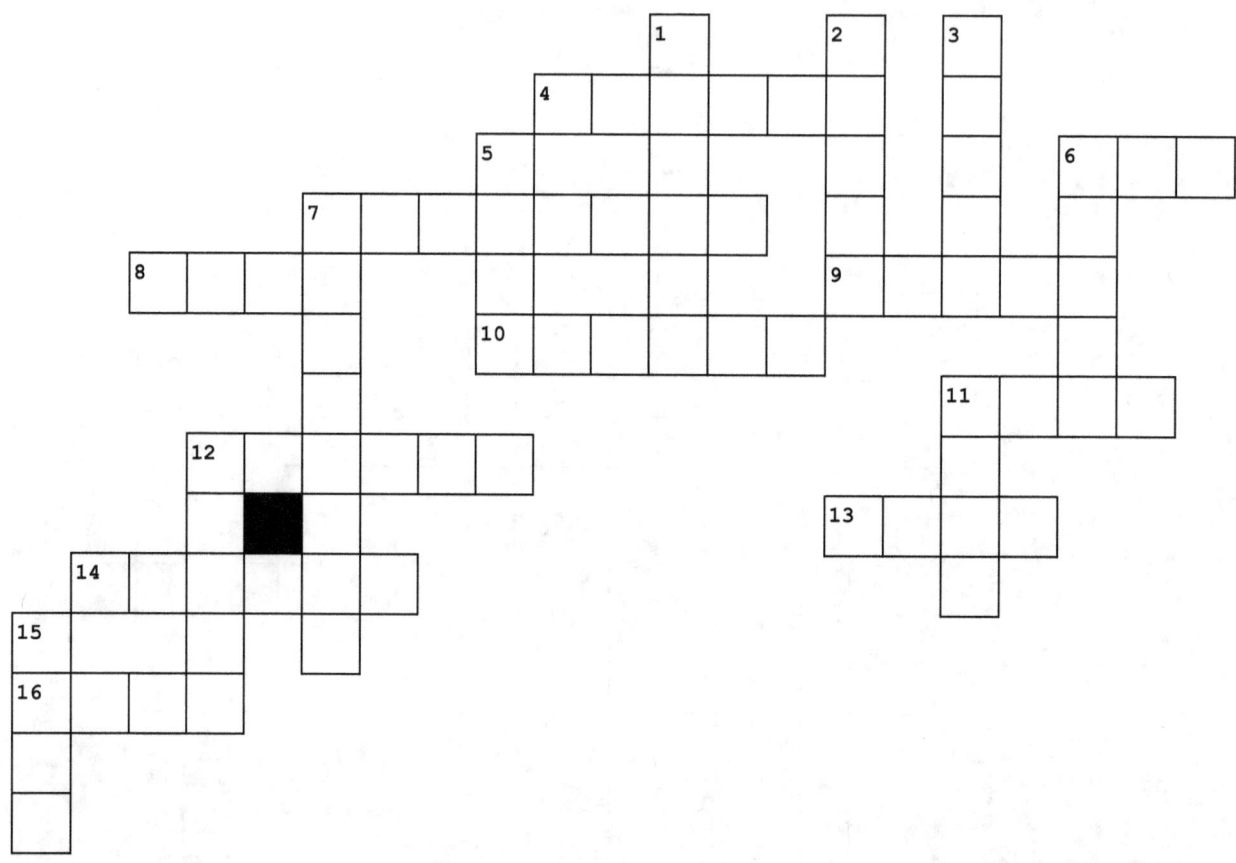

Across
4. medical term meaning pregnant
6. medical term meaning stretch
7. medical term meaning appendix
8. medical term meaning inflammation
9. medical term meaning joints
10. medical term meaning inner chamber
11. medical term meaning fear
12. medical term meaning braid
13. medical term meaning light
14. medial term meaning ovary
16. medical term meaning flow

Down
1. medical term meaning upper jawbone
2. medical term meaning swelling
3. medical term meaning bud
5. medical term meaning slender
6. medical term meaning ankle
7. medical term meaning weakness
11. medical term meaning voice or sound
12. medical term meaning to eat
15. medical term meaning rainbow

NCLEX-3

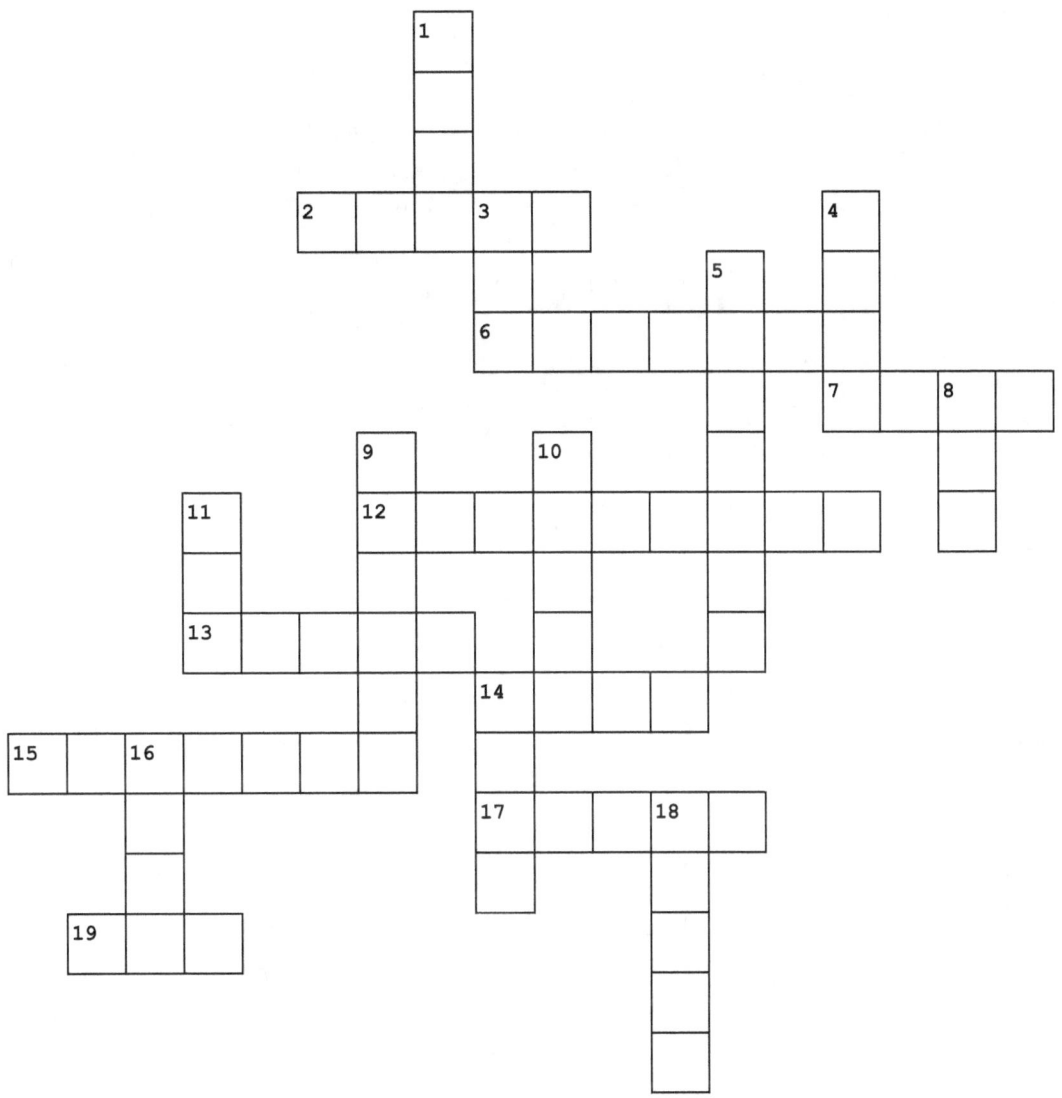

Across
2. Meaning of the medical root staphyl
6. Meaning of the medical root kary-
7. Medical term for a cutting instrument
12. Meaning of the suffix -plegia
13. Meaning of the medical root for scale like
14. Meaning of the suffix phil, philia, philic
15. Meaning of the medical root schizo-, schiz
17. Meaning of the medical root men-
19. Meaning of the medical root pnea-

Down
1. Medical term for after, behind
3. Medical term meaning all, entire
4. Medical root for distance
5. Medical term for movement
8. Meaning of the medical root andr- or hom-
9. Meaning of the medical prefix ana-
10. Medical term for edge of the eyelid
11. Meaning of the medical prefix pyo-
14. Medical term for Loins
16. Medical term for alive
18. Medical term for swift, rapid

NCLEX-4

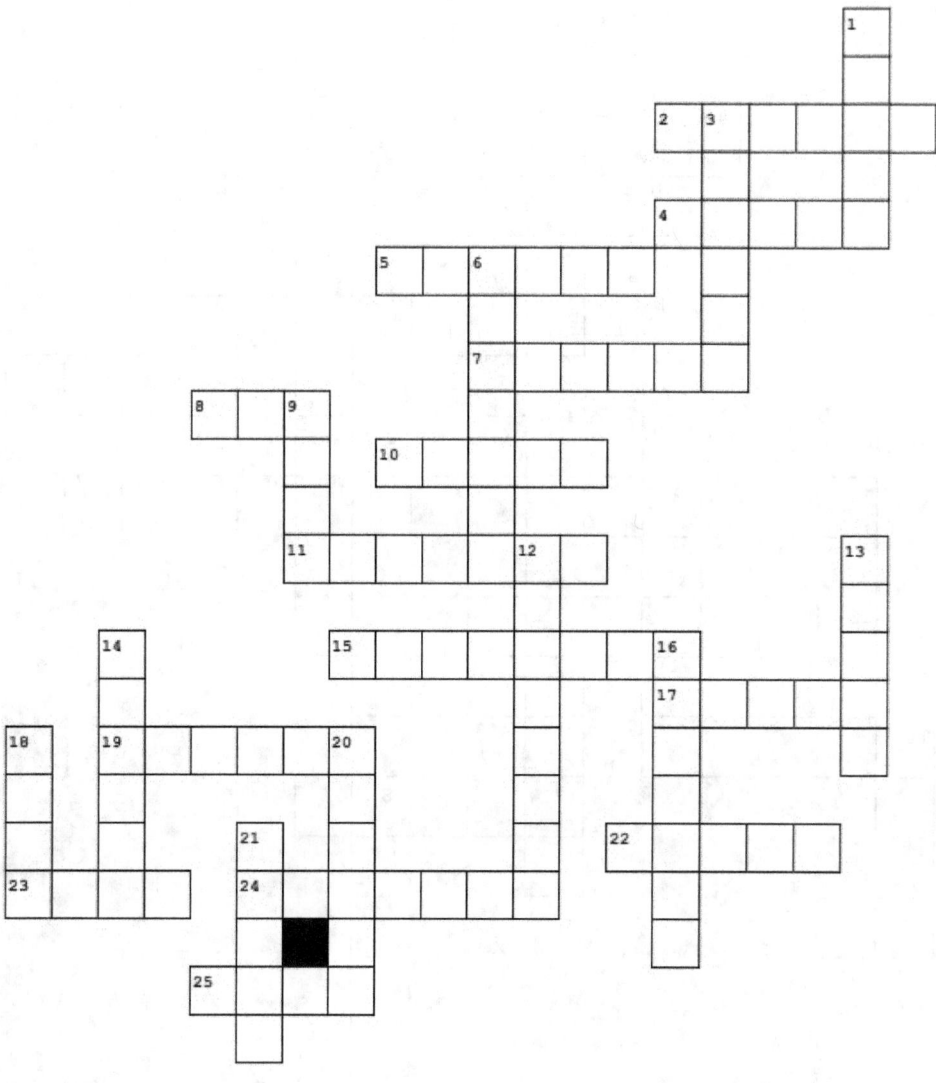

Across
2. Medical term for Reno
4. Arthro
5. Medical term for Pertaining to blood
7. Term for White
8. Medical term for Complains of
10. surrounding or around
11. Term for Gastro
15. Medical term for term for adrenal glands
17. instrument for visual examination
19. Medical term for Surgical removal
22. Pertaining to blood or lymph vessels
23. Medical term for Bad difficult or painful
24. Medical term for Rapture
25. Term for New

Down
1. term for thoraco
3. Medical term for Surgical incision
6. Medical term for Abnormal softening
9. Medical term for Abnormal condition
12. Medical term for Surgical procedure to remove fluid
13. Term for Excessive or to increase
14. Term for Hystero
16. Surgical creation of an opening
18. term for cephalo
20. Medical term for Fast or rapid
21. Medical term for Abnormal flow

NCLEX-5

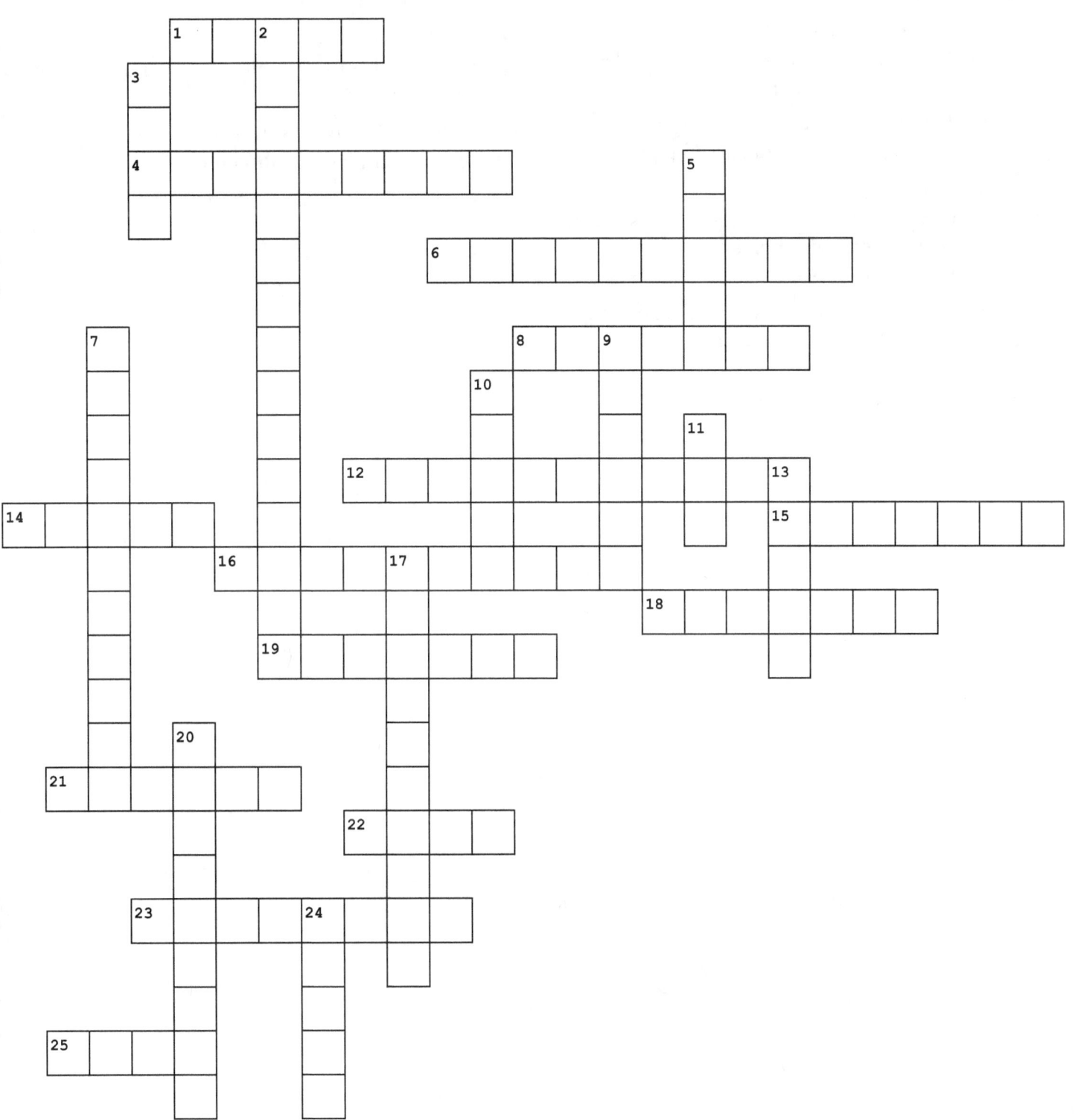

Across
1. Medical terminology for Cardi
4. Medical meaning for pneumon
6. The ability to adapt, cope, and recover from adversity or stress.

Down
2. Medical terminology for hardening
3. Medical meaning for derm
5. Medical terminology for steth

8. medical meaning of spir
12. A school of psychology that focuses on observable behavior and emphasizes the role of environment in shaping behavior.
14. Medical meaning for sphygm
15. An unpleasant emotional state characterized by feelings of fear, worry, and unease.
16. study of human behavior
18. Eating disorder known as Binge eating
19. Medical meaning for gastro
21. A physiological and psychological response to environmental demands or pressure.
22. medical meaning of oste
23. Eating disorder which a person have abnormally low body weight and intense fear of gaining weight- ANOREXIA
25. Medical terminology for below

7. The process of growth, maturation, and change that occurs throughout the lifespan.
9. Medical terminology for remove
10. Medical meaning of brach
11. Medical meaning for cost
13. having high energy, excitement over a sustained period of time
17. protein in red blood cells that carries oxygen
20. Medical terminology for tooth
24. Medical terminology for swelling

NCLEX-6

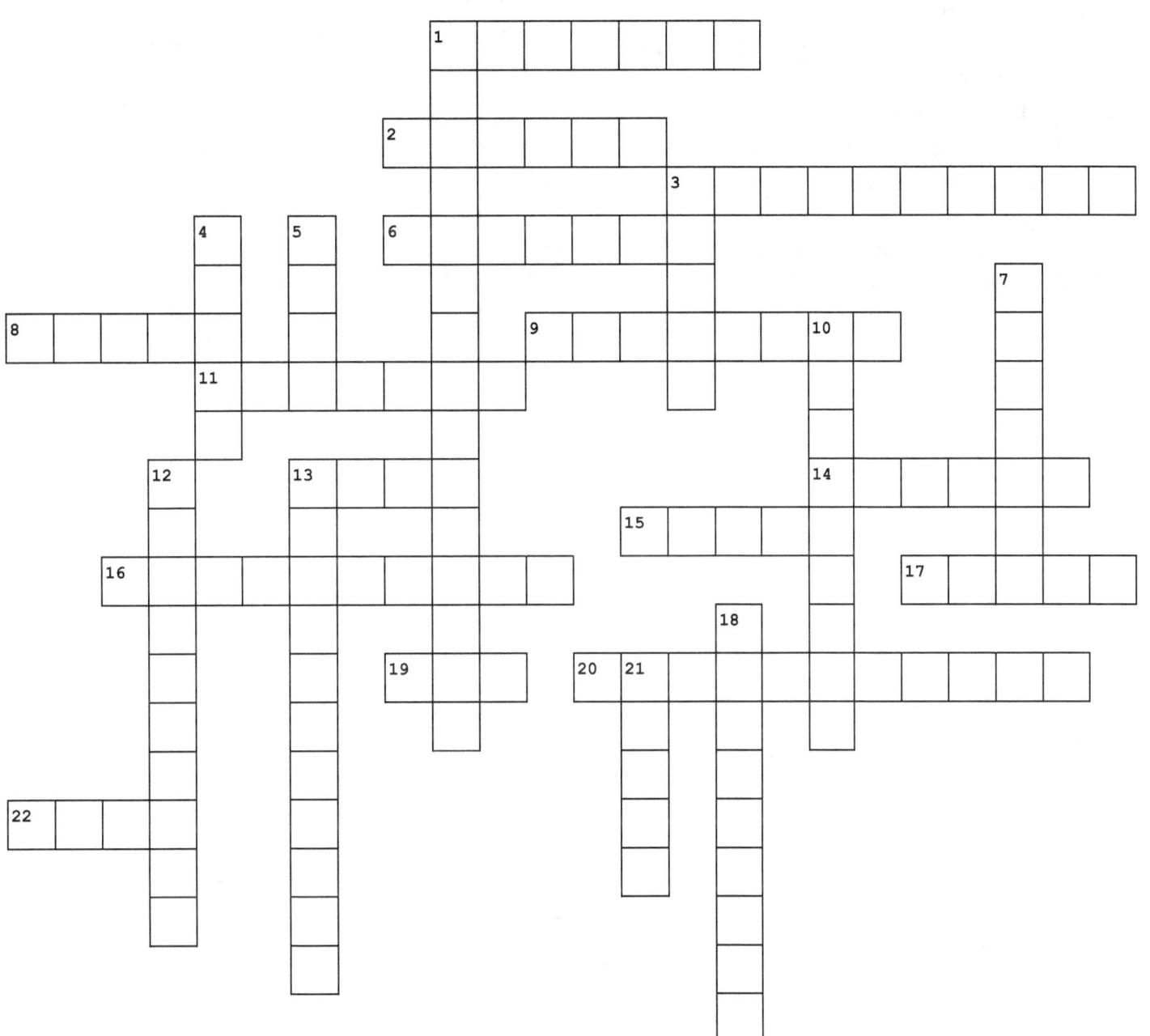

Across

1. An unpleasant emotional state characterized by feelings of fear, worry, and unease.
2. A physiological and psychological response to environmental demands or pressure.
3. protein in red blood cells that carries oxygen
6. medical meaning of spir
8. Medical meaning for sphygm
9. Eating disorder which a person have abnormally low body weight and intense fear of gaining

Down

1. Medical terminology for hardening
3. Medical terminology for Cardi
4. Medical terminology for steth
5. Medical terminology for below
7. Eating disorder known as Binge eating
10. Medical meaning for pneumon
12. The ability to adapt, cope, and recover from adversity or stress.

weight
11. Medical meaning for gastro
13. medical meaning of oste
14. Medical terminology for remove
15. having high energy, excitement over a sustained period of time
16. study of human behavior
17. Medical meaning of brach
19. Medical meaning for cost
20. The process of growth, maturation, and change that occurs throughout the lifespan.
22. Medical meaning for derm

13. A school of psychology that focuses on observable behavior and emphasizes the role of environment in shaping behavior.
18. Medical terminology for tooth
21. Medical terminology for swelling

NCLEX-7

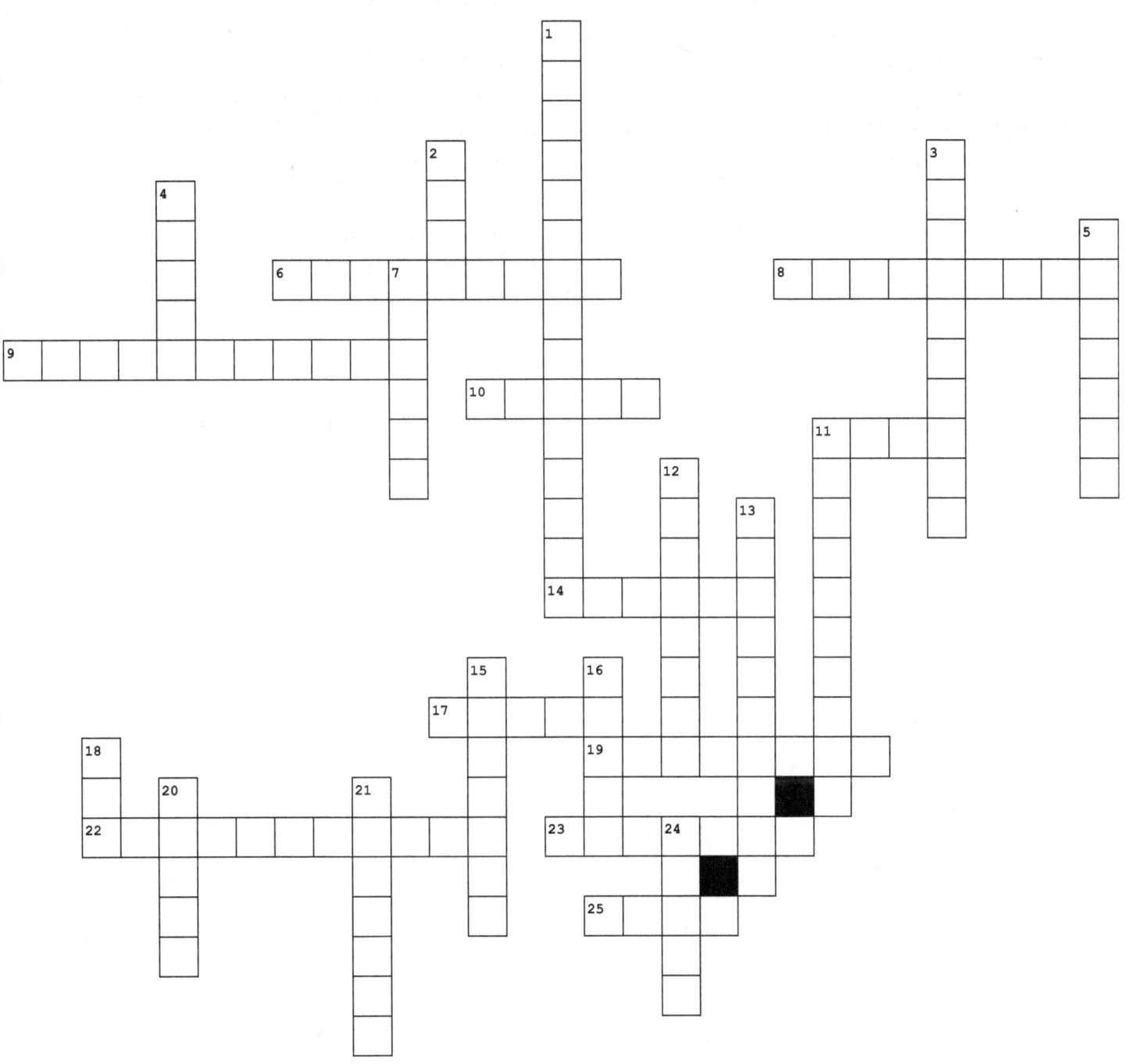

Across

6. Medical terminology for tooth
8. Medical meaning for pneumon
9. The process of growth, maturation, and change that occurs throughout the lifespan.
10. Medical terminology for swelling
11. Medical terminology for below
14. A physiological and psychological response to environmental demands or pressure.

Down

1. Medical terminology for hardening
2. Medical meaning for derm
3. study of human behavior
4. Medical meaning of brach
5. An unpleasant emotional state characterized by feelings of fear, worry, and unease.
7. Medical terminology for remove

17. Medical meaning for sphygm
19. Eating disorder which a person have abnormally low body weight and intense fear of gaining weight
22. A school of psychology that focuses on observable behavior and emphasizes the role of environment in shaping behavior.
23. Medical meaning for gastro
25. medical meaning of oste

11. protein in red blood cells that carries oxygen
12. The part of the mind that represents internalized societal rules and values, according to Freud's psychoanalytic theory.
13. The ability to adapt, cope, and recover from adversity or stress.
15. Eating disorder known as Binge eating
16. Medical terminology for Cardi
18. Medical meaning for cost
20. Medical terminology for steth
21. medical meaning of spir
24. having high energy, excitement over a sustained period of time

NCLEX-8

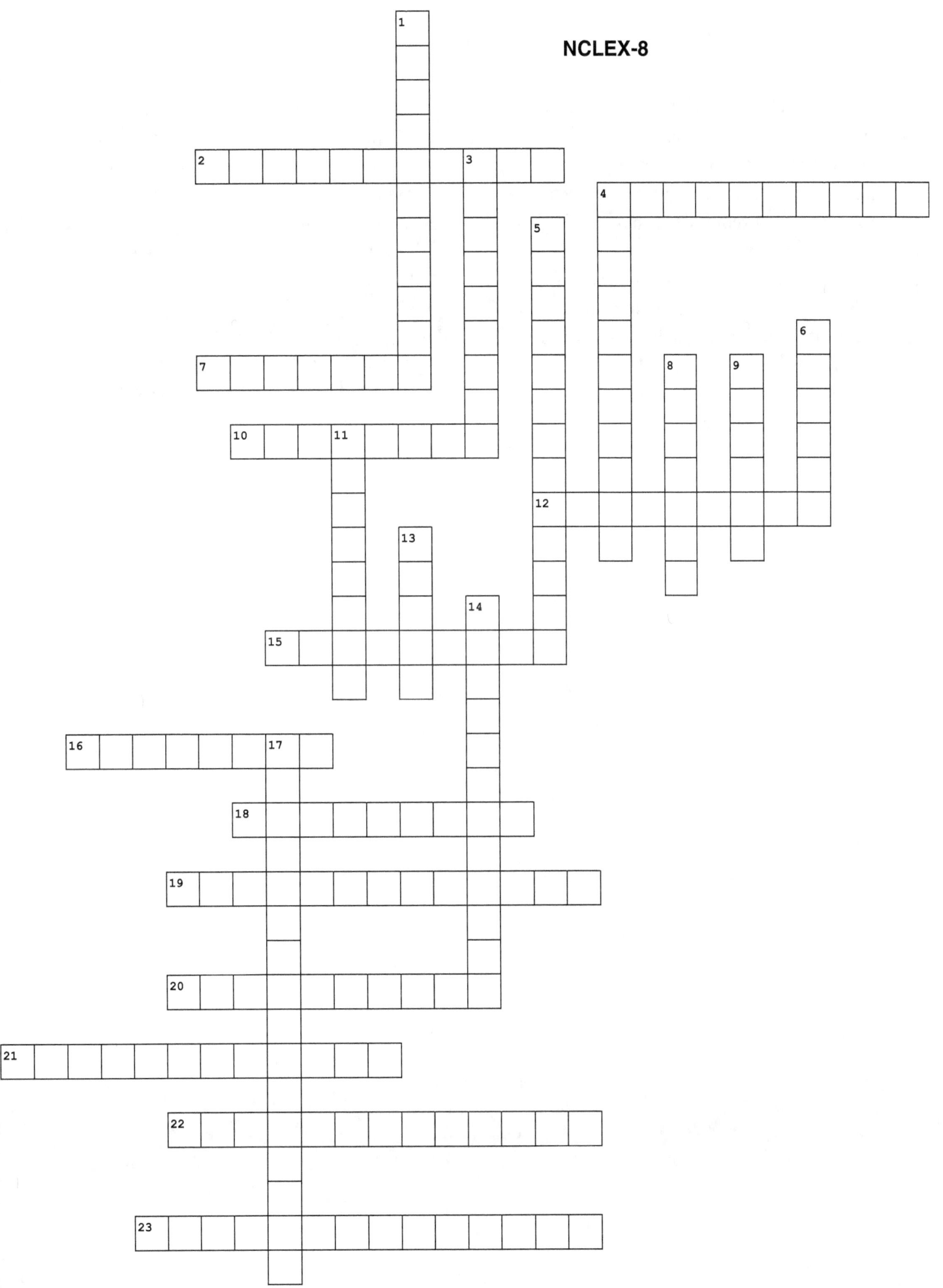

Across

2. Protein in red blood cells that carries oxygen
4. Medical terminology for fast breathing
7. Disease caused by lack of Vitamin C:
10. Gland in your neck that regulate your metabolism
12. Person with recurrent seizures has _____
15. Medical condition that causes high blood sugar
16. Disease caused by Mosquitoes bites in Africa
18. Medical terminology for excessive urination
19. Medical terminology for high blood pressure
20. Hormone that helps you fall asleep
21. Medical terminology for low potassium
22. Specialist doctor for the heart
23. Specialist doctor for the skin

Down

1. Medical terminology for white blood cells
3. Medical terminology for inability to sleep
4. ,Medical terminology for fast heart rate
5. Medical terminology for low blood sugar .
6. Medical terminology for the kidney
8. Infection you may get after bat bite
9. Condition that causes the salivary gland to swell up
11. Virus that causes German measles
13. Infection you may get after Tick bite
14. Medical terminology for low body water
17. terminology for loss of appetite for food

NCLEX-9

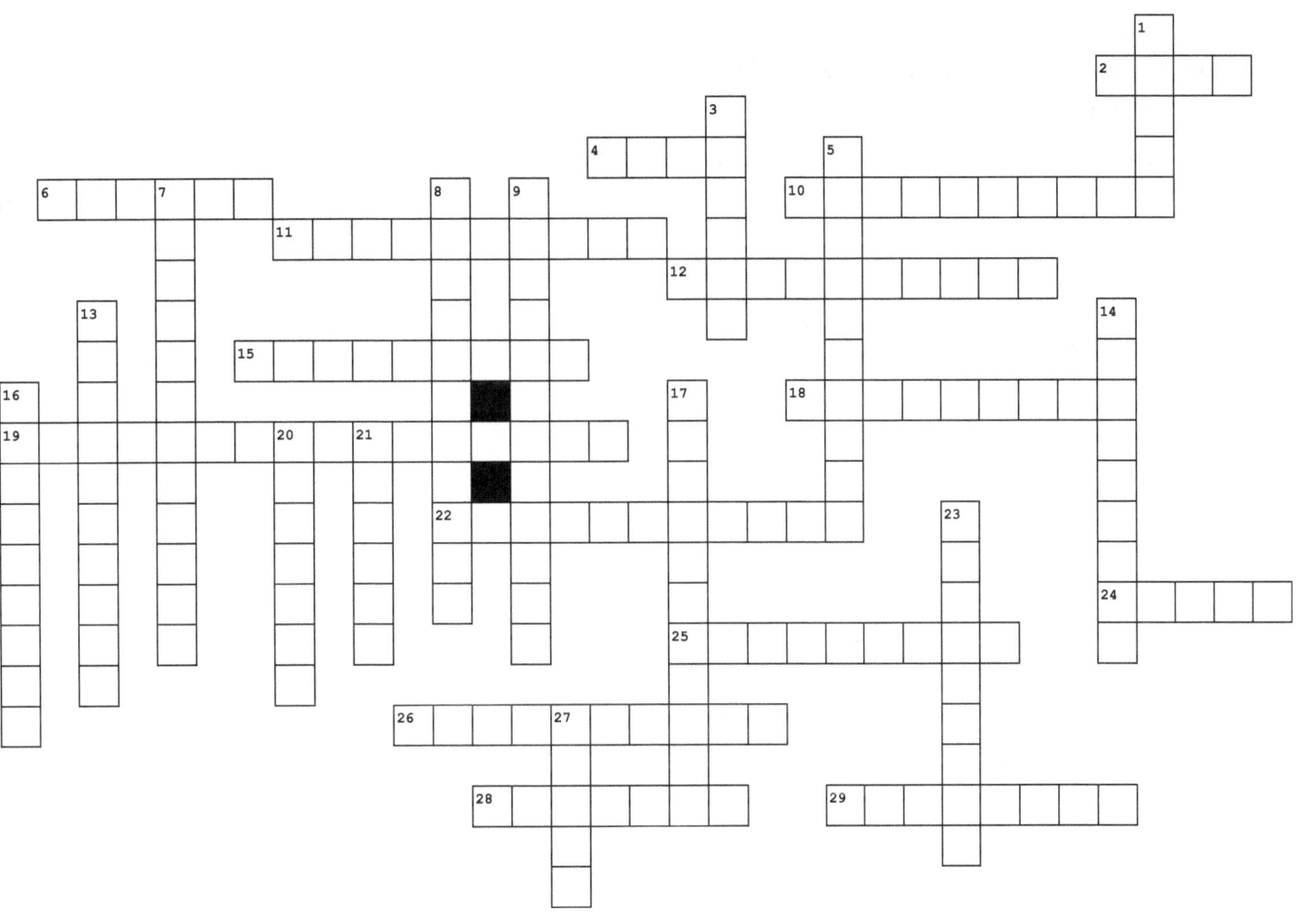

Across

2. A piece of clothing that covers most of the body of a patient.
4. A person's skeleton consists of ...
6. A piece of an organ, a little blood, etc.
10. A part of a hospital where a particular type of treatment is provided.
11. Department where healthcare for pregnant women is provided.
12. Department where heart diseases are treated.
15. When a woman is about to have a baby.
18. The manner of treating a patient.
19. He/she performs surgery pain relief and preparation.
22. Department where you go, if you have problems with joints.

Down

1. A point where two bones meet in the body.
3. A pan used as a toilet by a person who is too ill to get out of bed.
5. Department where children are cared for.
7. I am a general ..., I know everything about general medicine
8. Department where skin cancer can be treated.
9. A written message from a doctor that officially tells someone to use a medicine, therapy, etc.
13. A chair with wheels that is used by people who cannot walk because they are disabled, sick, or injured.
14. Laboratory where the samples are tested.
16. Department where X-rays and CT-scans are made for hospital departments.
17. Not safe.

24. A cotton fabric used to cover wounds or surgical incisions.
25. Department where there are a lot of patients in life-threatening condition.
26. Jane is a lab ... .
28. A device used for injecting liquids into the body.
29. It fills prescriptions.

20. Department where organ transplants are carried out.
21. A chemical that is found in the air, that has no color, taste, or smell, and that is necessary for life.
23. Method, operation, surgery.
27. I have the nursing schedules.

NCLEX-10

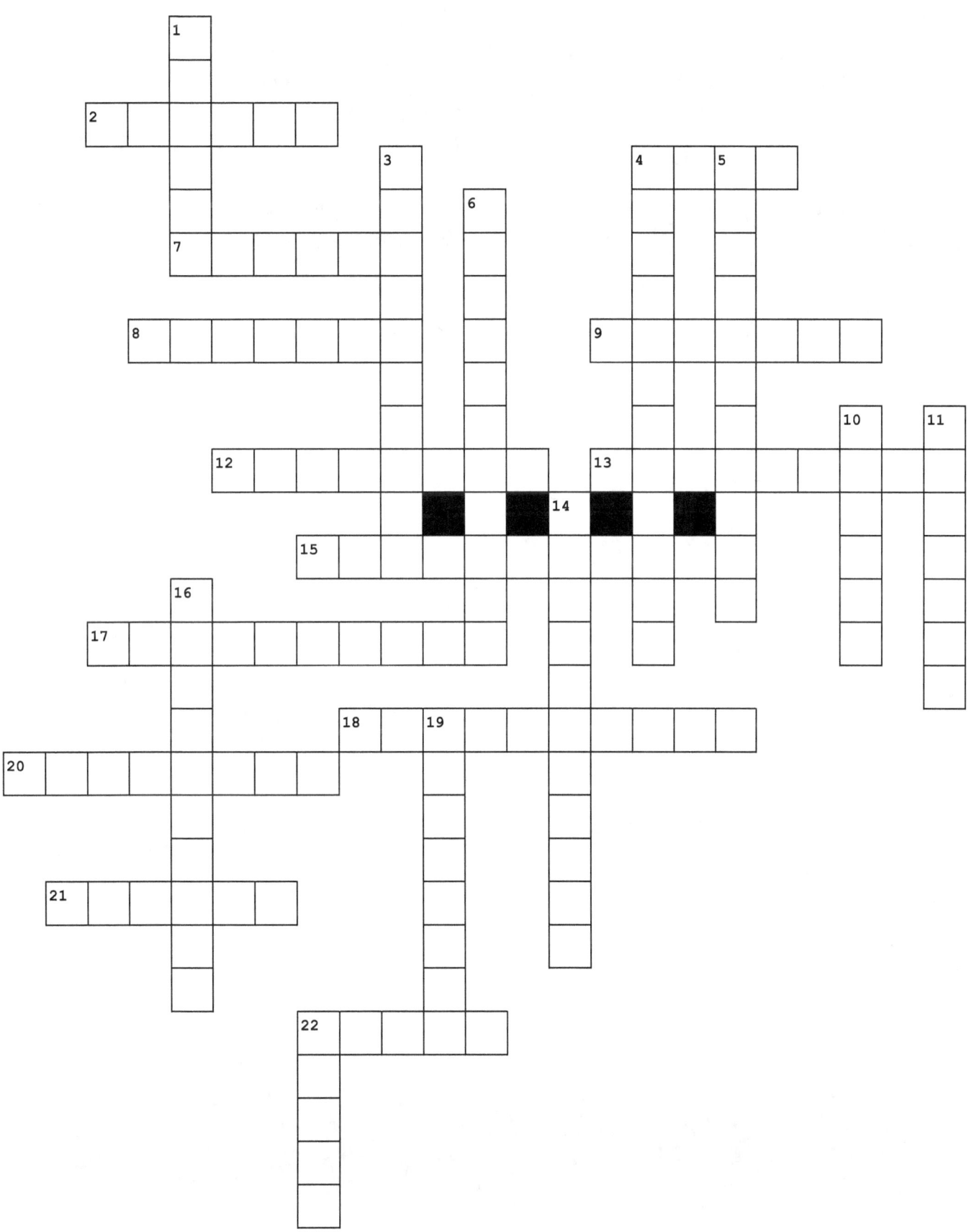

Across
2. towards
4. blue
7. toxin
8. kneecap
9. relating to eating
12. surgery
13. front
15. study of bones
17. mental disorders
18. doctor for children
20. eye doctor
21. vein
22. black

Down
1. away from
3. foot doctor
4. heart doctor
5. administers anesthesia
6. related to breathing
10. fingers and toes
11. urine
14. study and treatment of skin
16. study of women organs
19. memory loss
22. small

NCLEX-11

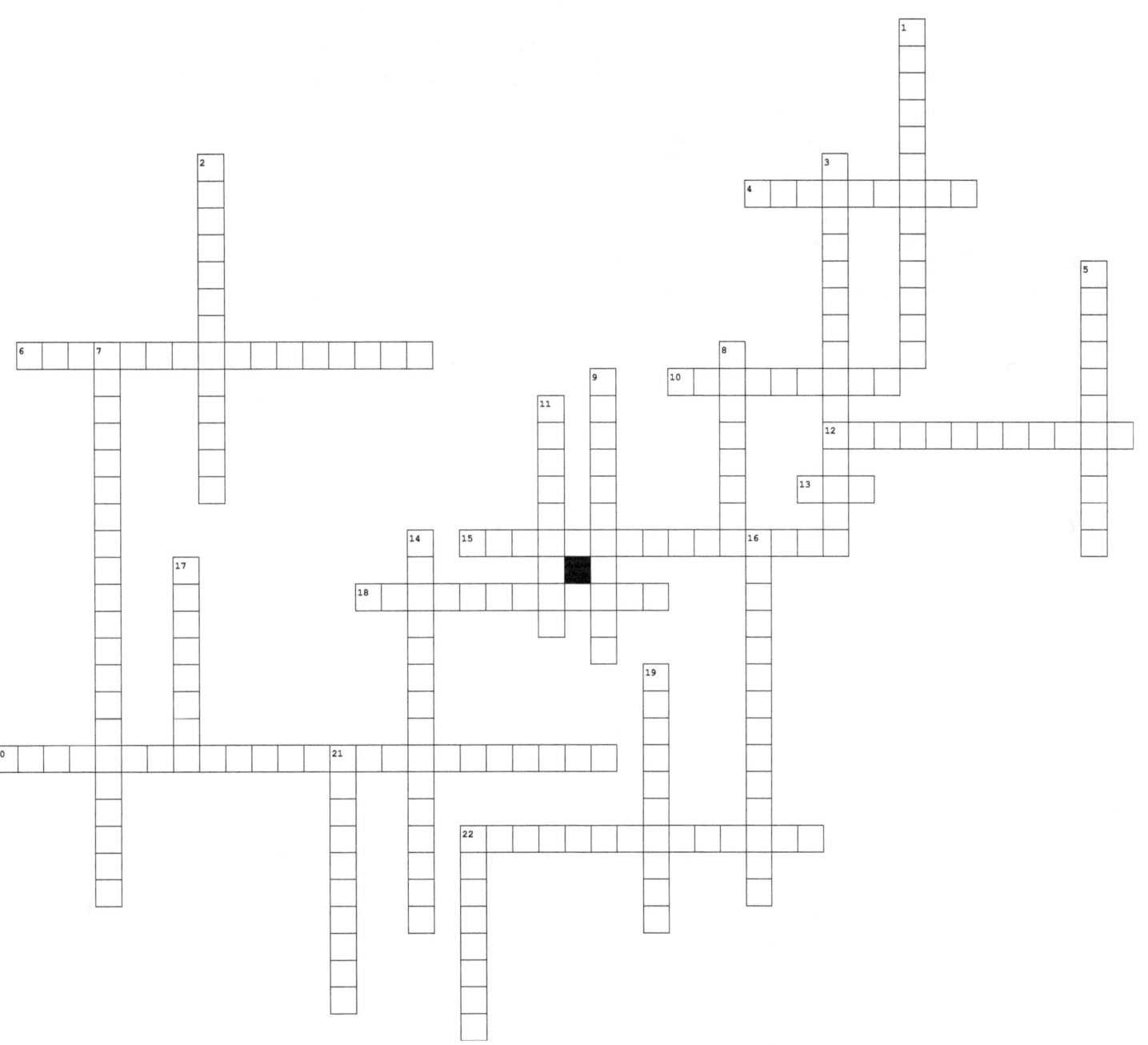

Across

4. increases urinary output
6. reduces heartbeat rate
10. suppress appetite
12. suppresses coughing
13. Man's best friend
15. prevents convulsions
18. reduces fever
20. treat muscle/bone condition

Down

1. relives tension
2. treats anemia
3. promotes easier breathing
5. stops vomiting
7. treat shock and drug poisoning
8. treats hormonal disorders/cancer
9. fight infection
11. promotes sleep

22. relives cold

14. elevate mood
16. slow blood-clotting process
17. supplements
19. promotes evacuation of bowels
21. relieve pain
22. neutralize stomach acid

NCLEX-12

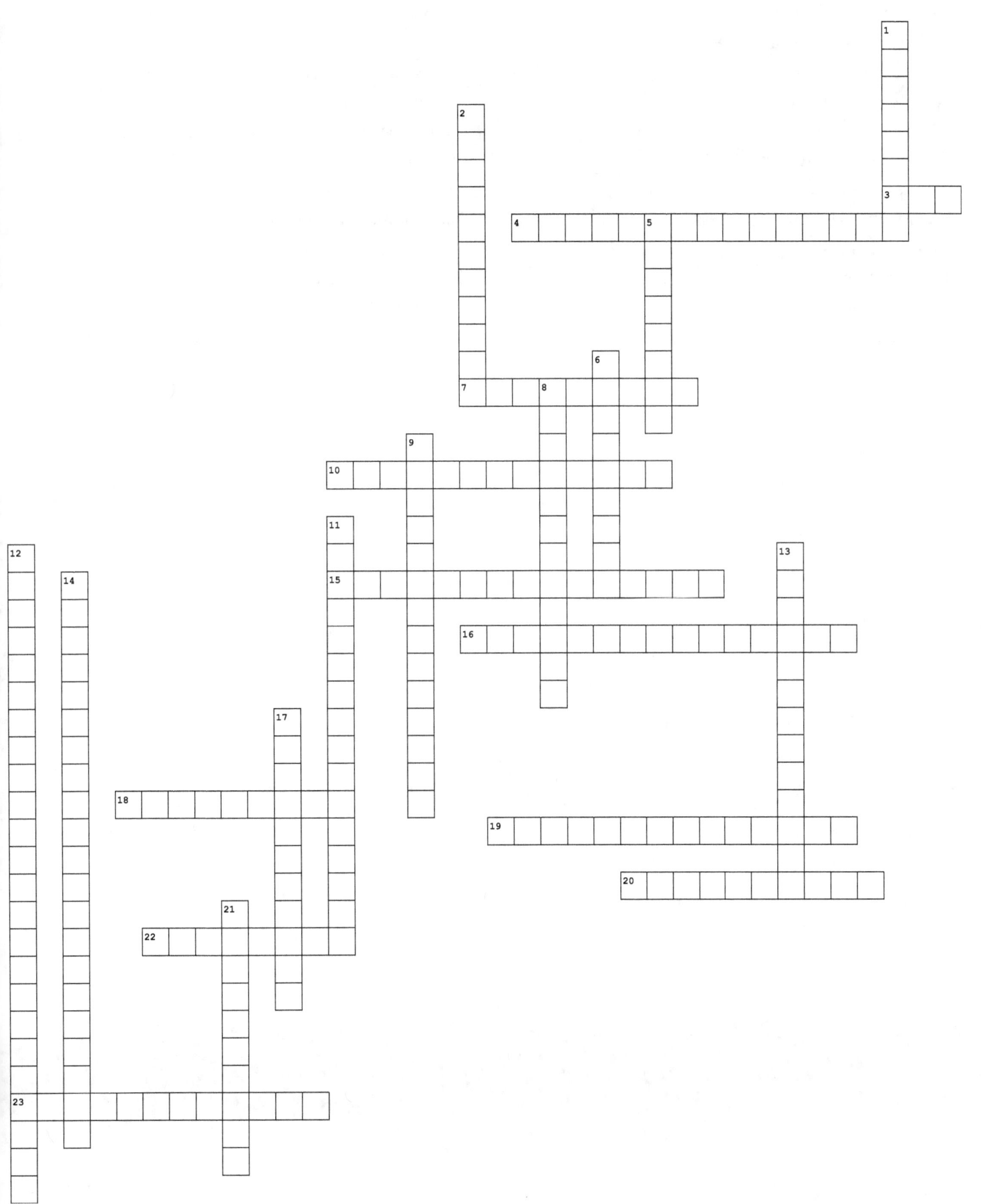

Across
3. Man's best friend
4. promotes easier breathing
7. promotes sleep
10. relives tension
15. elevate mood
16. prevents convulsions
18. suppress appetite
19. slow blood-clotting process
20. relieve pain
22. supplements
23. suppresses coughing

Down
1. neutralize stomach acid
2. stops vomiting
5. treats hormonal disorders/cancer
6. increases urinary output
8. reduces fever
9. relives cold
11. reduces heartbeat rate
12. treat muscle/bone condition
13. treats anemia
14. treat shock and drug poisoning
17. fight infection
21. promotes evacuation of bowels

NCLEX-13

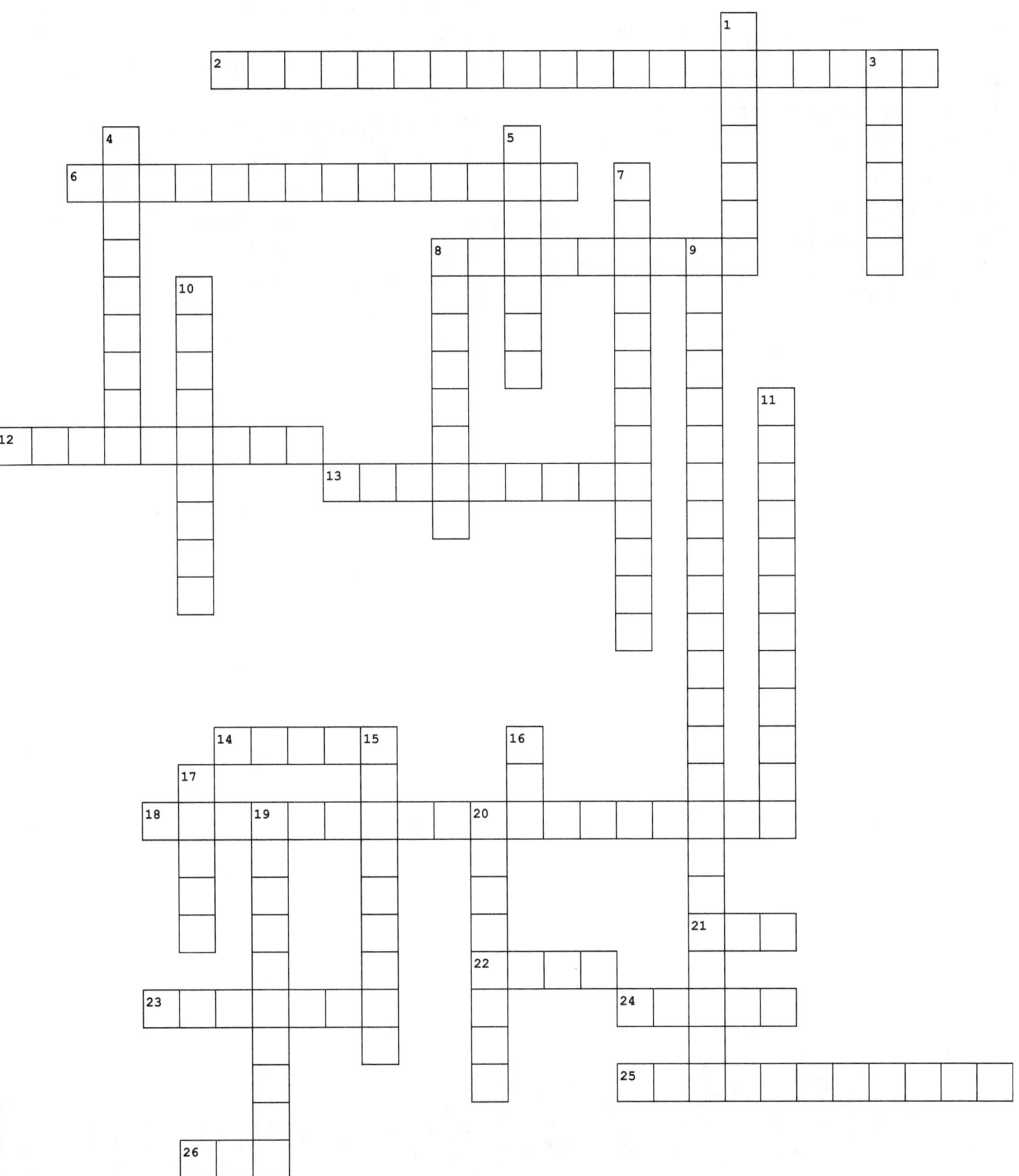

2. when a part of the heart muscle doesn't get enough blood
6. the pressure in the arteries when the heart rests between beats
8. infection of one or both of the lungs caused by bacteria, viruses, or fungi
12. ventilation breathing is defined as
13. the rate at which the heart beats
14. which bronchi is larger
18. the posterior tibial pulse
21. how many years to become Resp. Therapist
22. air blockage and breathing problems
23. two large tubes that carry air from your windpipe to your lungs
24. result for kinesiology is the study of
25. mechanics of human movement and how they impact our health and wellbeing
26. Favorite Respiratory therapist

1. one of the conducting airways
3. how do we breath
4. most important muscle used for breathing
5. one of the Covid vaccines
7. how many bones in our body
8. inflammation or irritation of the lining of the lungs and chest
9. Up to 49 percent of chest pain comes from what
10. breathing cycle is controlled by the
11. walls enclose this cavity and its structures
15. how many weeks lung therapy
16. causes scarring of the lung
17. Symptom of pnuemonia
19. how many muscles in our body
20. for the lungs

NCLEX-15

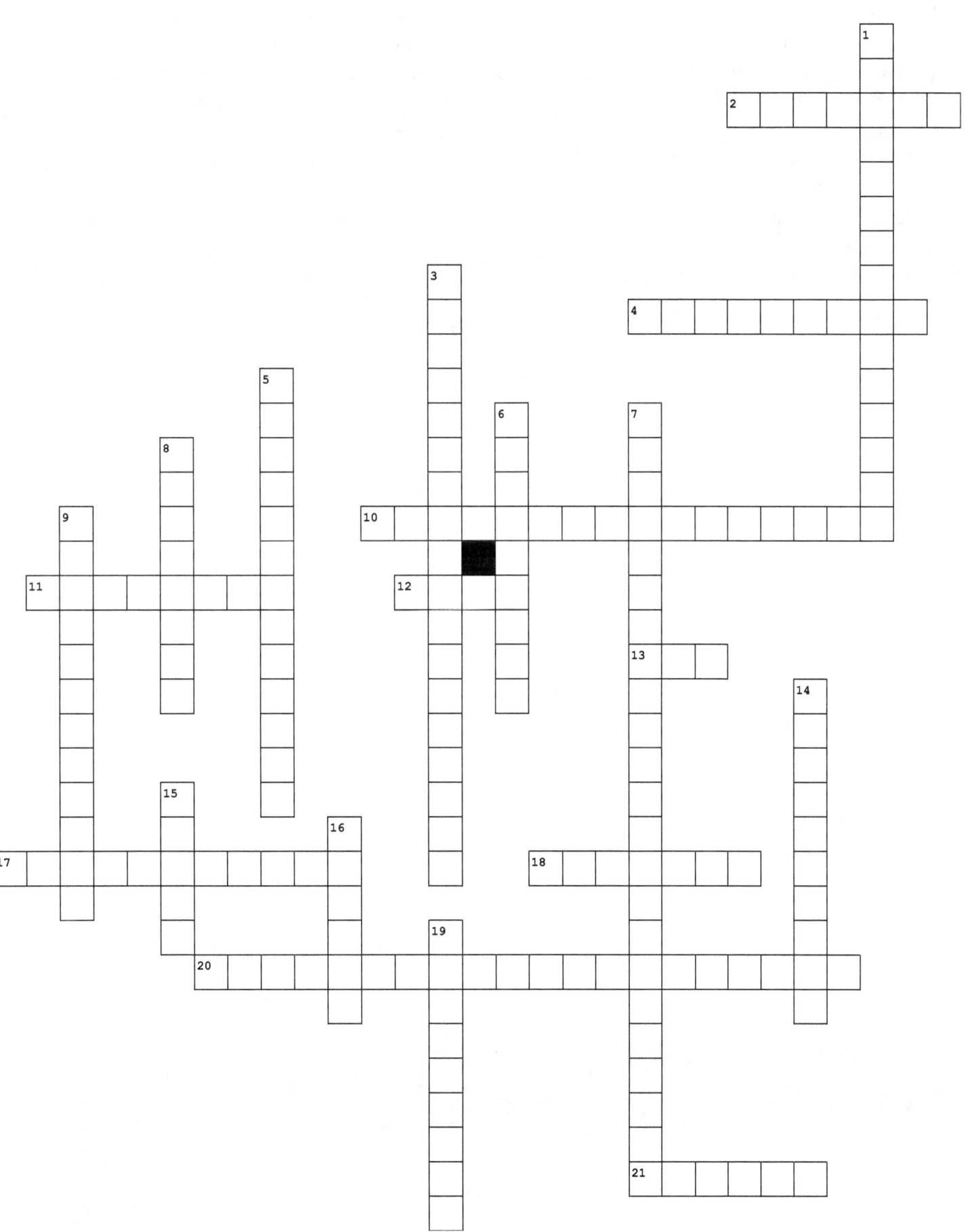

Across

2. Three copies of a chromosome
4. Indication of UTI
10. a cancer treatment that uses high doses of radiation to kill cancer cells and shrink tumors (2 words)
11. Broken bone
12. What syndrome is treated with salt
13. nothing by mouth
17. Health maintenance screening
18. Kneecap
20. Medical emergency in diabetics (two words)
21. an overgrowth of scar tissue that can form after surgery or an injury

Down

1. Removal of gallbladder
3. Scan of the abdomen
5. A prenatal test that can diagnose genetic disorders
6. This med should never be pushed IV
7. Mini-stroke (3 words)
8. The cessation of electrical and mechanical activity of the heart
9. Enlarged Heart
14. Stinky feet
15. The only bone in the human body not attached to another bone
16. prefix for uterus
19. Region of the brain in charge of vision

NCLEX-14

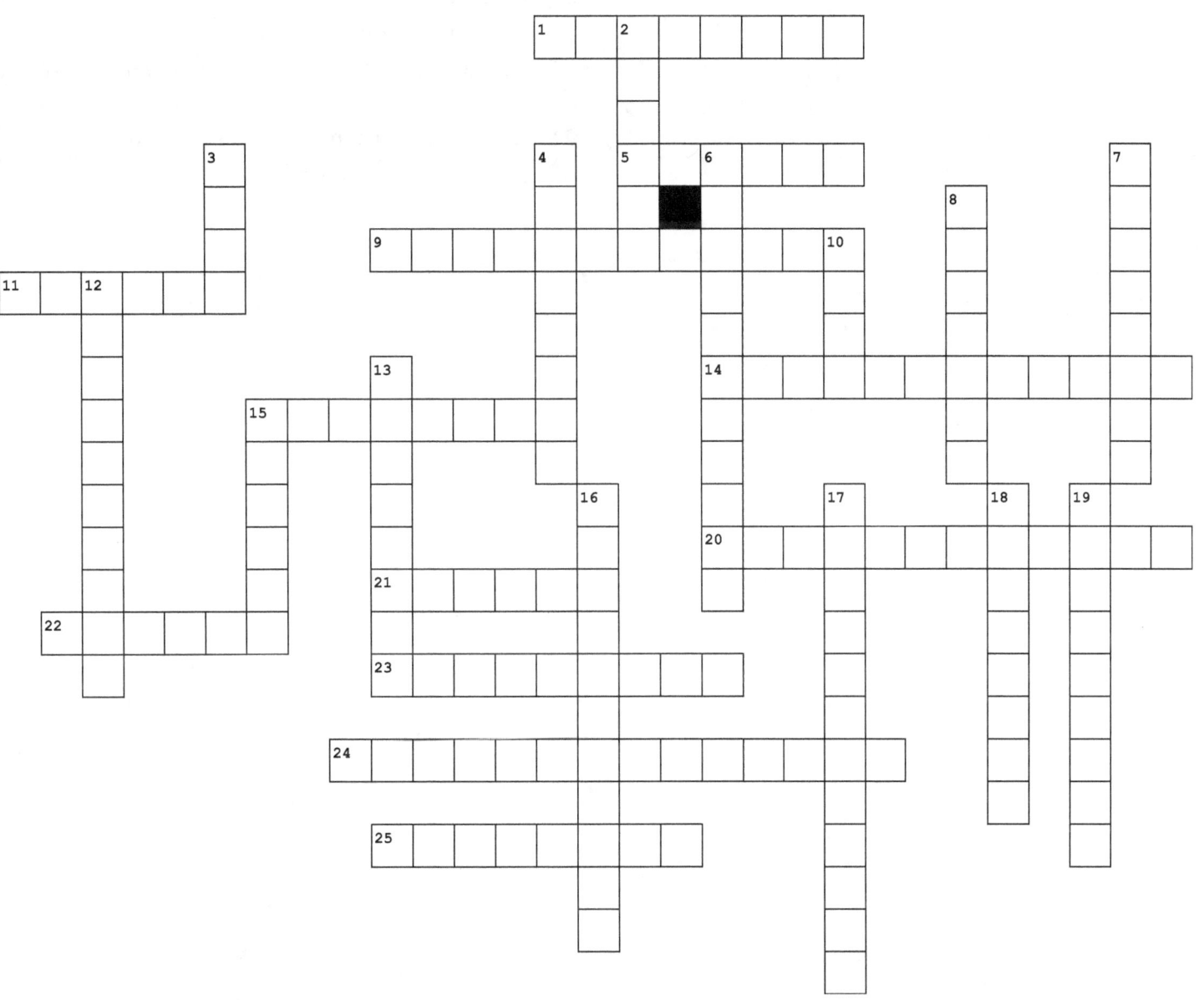

Across

1. Medical term that means ringing in the ears
5. Word root meaning "liver"
9. Medical term that means painful menstruation
11. Medical term that means a hair follicle that is plugged with sebum i.e. blackhead, white head
14. Medical term that means loss of bone density
15. Term meaning "above"
20. Medical term for sleep walking
21. Angioma Medical term that means a small blood vessel tumor
22. Word root meaning "heart"

Down

2. Wood root meaning "kidney"
3. Prefix meaning "in or inside"
4. Wood root meaning "eyelid"
6. Medical term that means the involuntary contraction of the diaphragm; street name is hiccups
7. Medical term that means excessive growth of facial and body hair in women
8. Word root that means "lungs"
10. Prefix meaning "before"
12. Infarction Medical term that means death of heart

23. Wood root meaning "brain"
24. Medical term for ovarian cysts
25. Word root meaning "vertebra"

muscle tissue; street name is heart attack
13. Medical term that means the beginning or first menstruation
15. Word root meaning "spleen"
16. Medical term for red blood cell
17. Medical term that means the inability to control urination
18. Medical term that means good digestion
19. Term meaning "both sides"

NCLEX-19

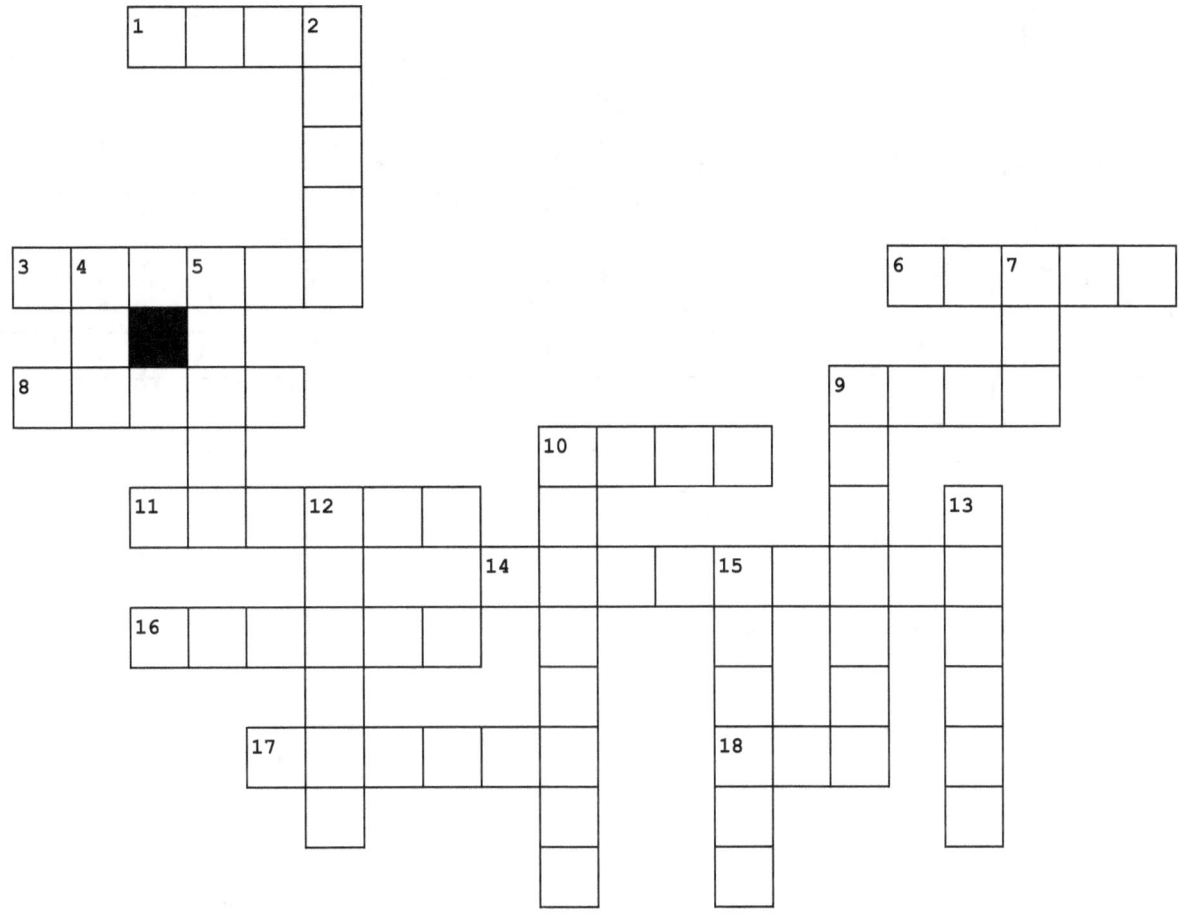

Across
1. vein
3. ear
6. hands
8. forhead
9. tooth
10. leg
11. lip
14. arm
16. blood
17. stomach
18. foot

Down
2. car
4. heart
5. tongue
7. nose
9. fingers
10. brain
12. neck
13. sholders
15. body

NCLEX-20

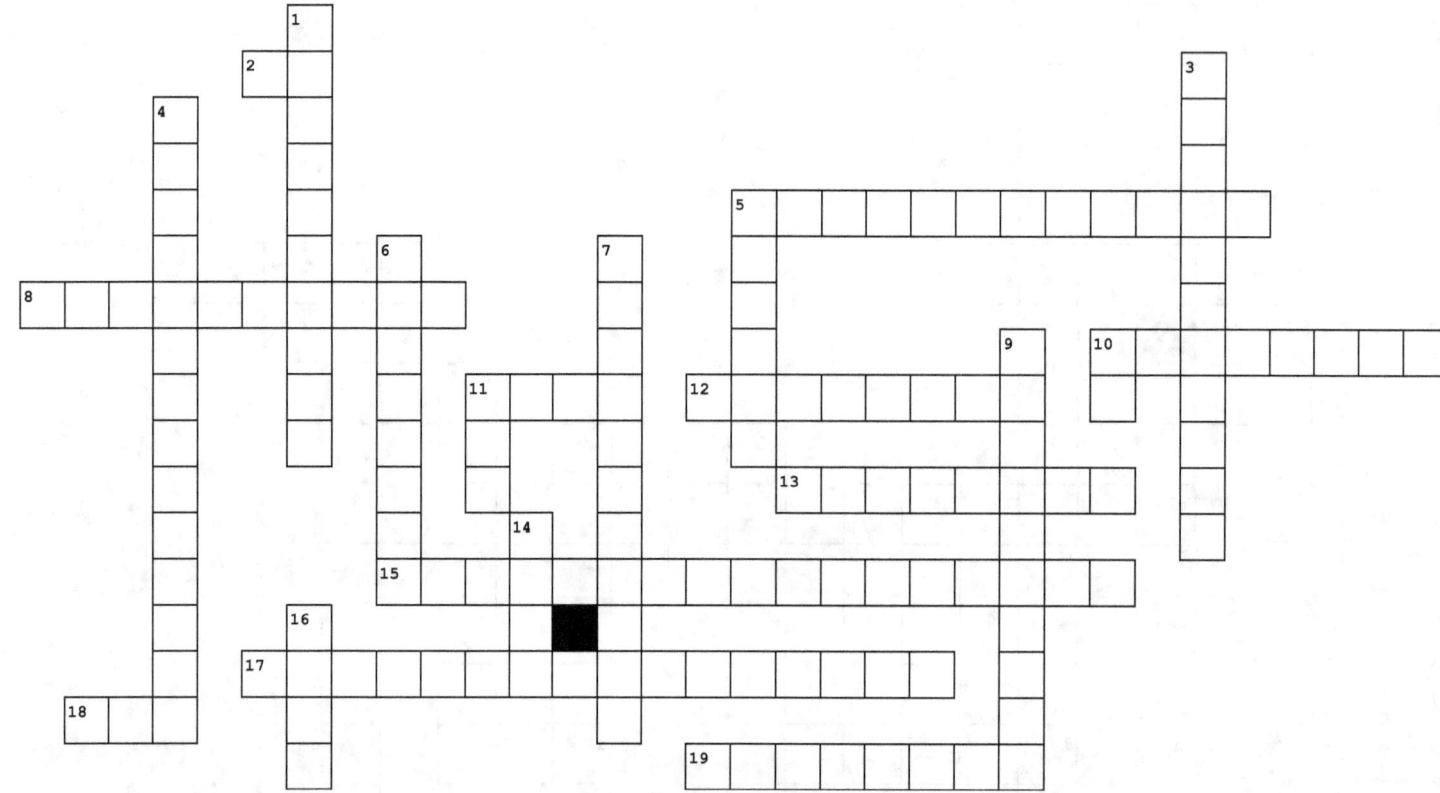

Across

2. blood pressure
5. high blood pressure as a result of pressure in a blood vessel
8. infarction heart attack
10. heart
11. top of the heart
12. artery the major blood vessels of the heart Cardiac arrest a complete stopping of the heart myocardial heart
13. chest
15. uses electricity to see parts of the cardiovascular system
17. used to measure blood pressure
18. beats per minute
19. an artery with a weakened wall

Down

1. outer layer of the heart
3. the layer of the heart chambers
4. uses sound to see parts of the cardiovascular system
5. blood
6. veins swollen and dilated veins
7. septum wall between the right and left atria
9. middle muscular layer of the heart that pumps blood
10. cardiovascular
11. blood
14. echocardiogram
16. bottom of the heart

NCLEX-21

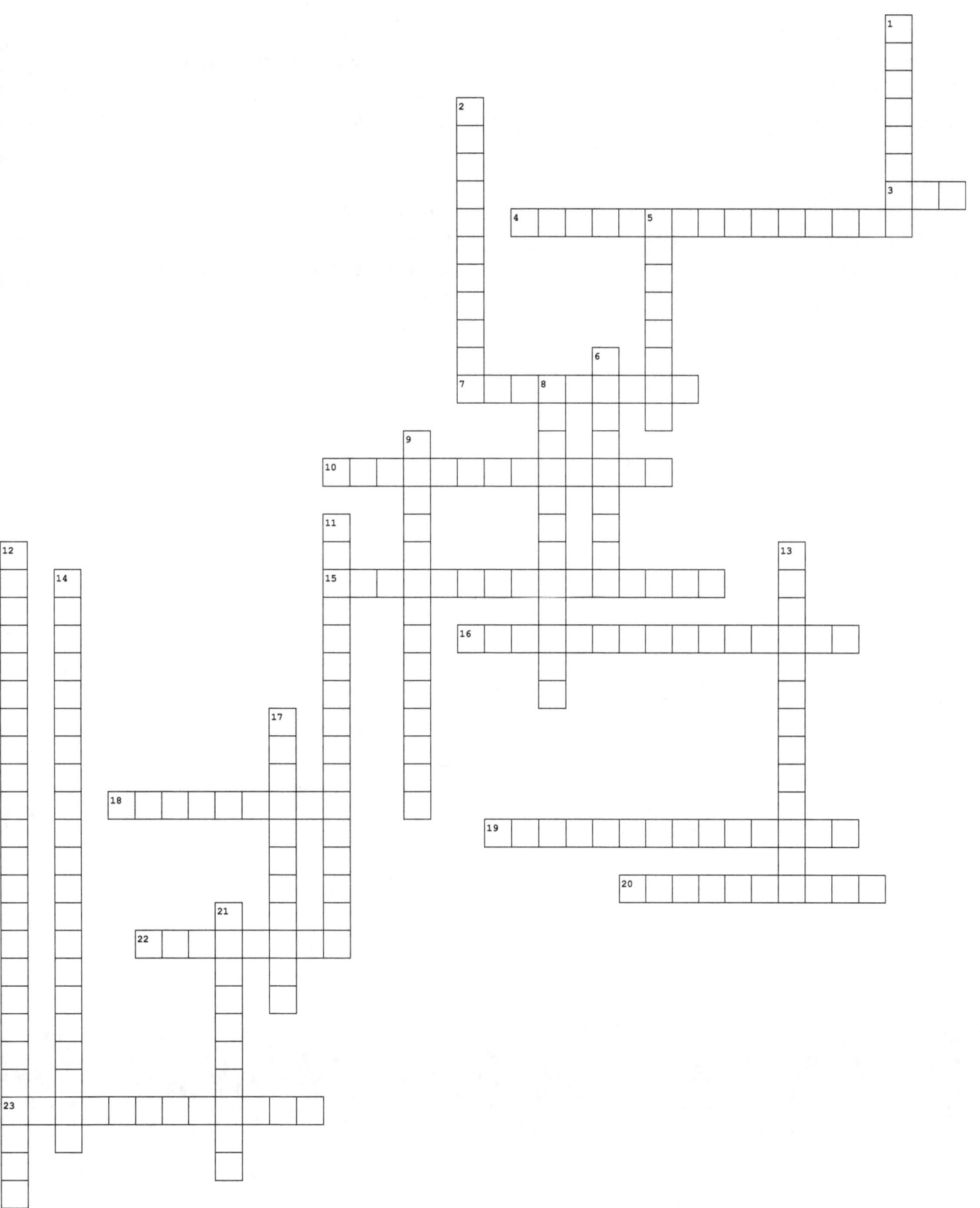

Across	**Down**
3. Man's best friend	1. neutralize stomach acid
4. promotes easier breathing	2. stops vomiting
7. promotes sleep	5. treats hormonal disorders/cancer
10. relives tension	6. increases urinary output
15. elevate mood	8. reduces fever
16. prevents convulsions	9. relives cold
18. suppress appetite	11. reduces heartbeat rate
19. slow blood-clotting process	12. treat muscle/bone condition
20. relieve pain	13. treats anemia
22. supplements	14. treat shock and drug poisoning
23. suppresses coughing	17. fight infection
	21. promotes evacuation of bowels

NCLEX-22

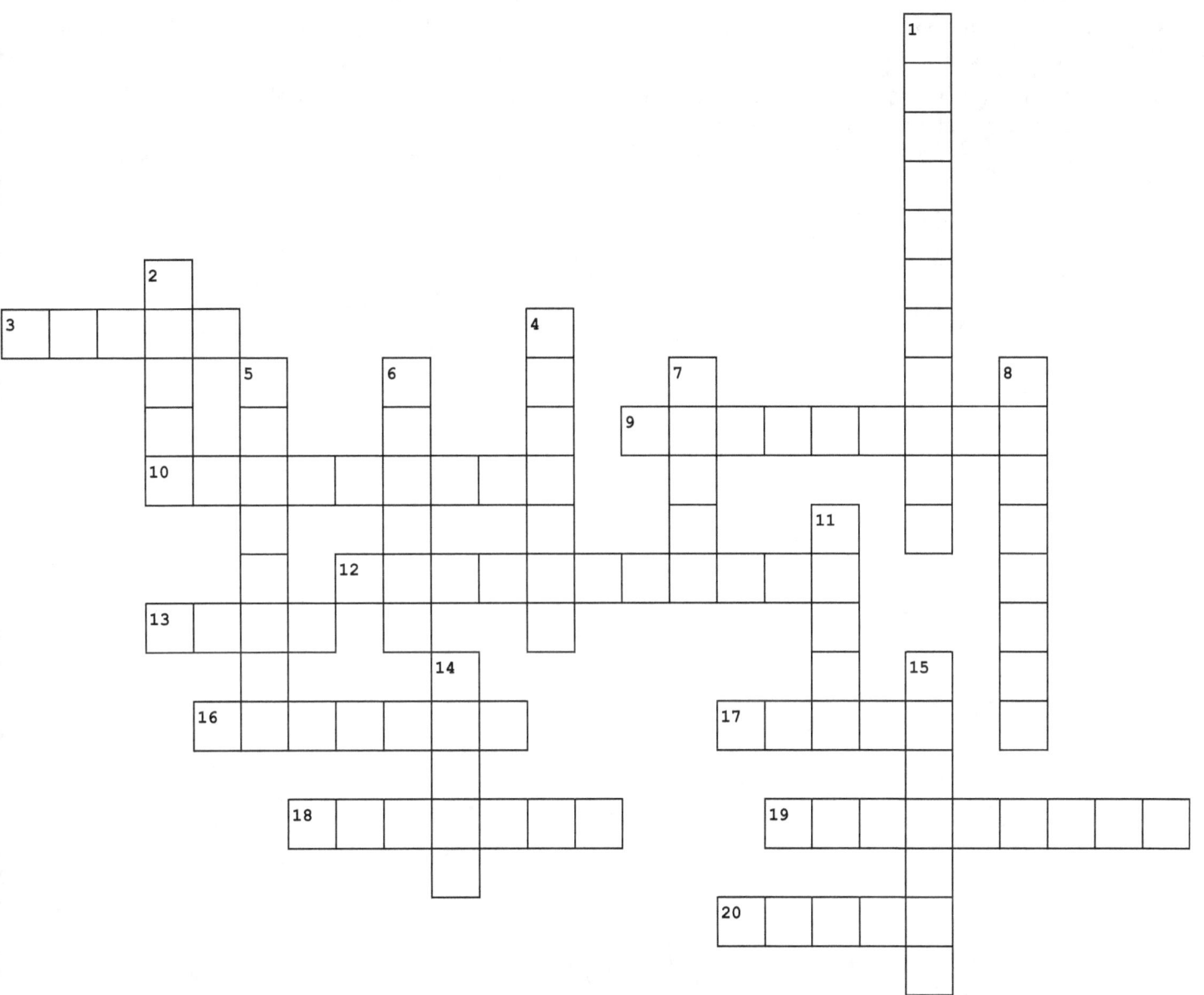

Across

3. the red liquid that circulates in the veins and arteries of humans and animals, carrying oxygen and nutrients throughout the body

9. to recommend the use of a medicine or treatment

10. the identification of a disease or medical condition through examination and testing

12. the degree of hotness or coldness of something, usually measured with a thermometer

13. a mark left on the skin after a wound has healed

16. a physical or mental feature that indicates a medical condition

Down

1. the administration of a vaccine to stimulate the immune system and prevent disease

2. an injury to the body, typically caused by cutting or tearing the skin

4. a material used to cover and protect wounds or broken bones

5. a place where medicines are prepared and sold

6. correct or suitable according to social norms or standards

7. to provide medical care or attention to someone who is ill or injured

17. a person trained to care for sick or injured people, especially in a hospital

18. a medical procedure getting into the body to repair or remove damaged tissue

19. a shot given with a needle, often to administer medicine or vaccines

20. things used as medication or for recreational purposes, often with negative side effects

8. pills or syrups used to treat or prevent illness or disease

11. an abnormally high body temperature, often a symptom of illness

14. a sudden throw of air from the lungs, often due to irritation or infection

15. another word for death; the end of life

NCLEX-24

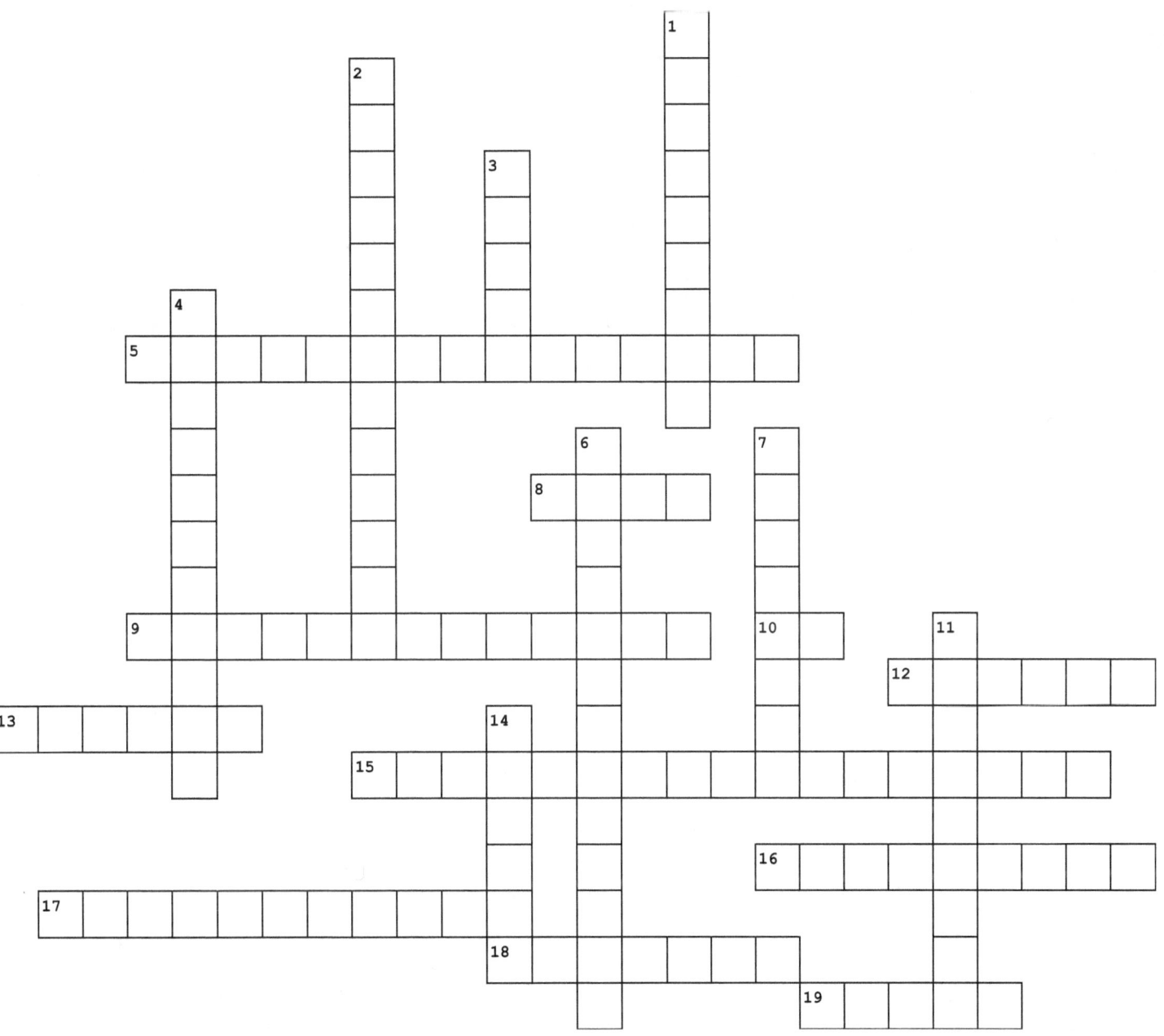

Across

5. Helps injured people improve their movement
8. A separate room/department in a hospital
9. Treats skin conditions
10. Where emergency health cases go by ambulance
12. diseases of the heart
13. An adjustable, wheeled stretcher
15. Used to detect heart problems
16. A department that performs x-rays
17. A device used to listen to the heart

Down

1. Identifying a present disease/illness
2. Treats blood conditions
3. Found in the wrist to count heartbeats
4. Used to take a patient's temperature
6. Treats babies and children
7. A device used to monitor oxygen levels
11. Predicting the course of a diagnosed illness
14. Used to weigh patient's

18. An instrument used to cut the skin
19. A qualified health care professional

NCLEX-25

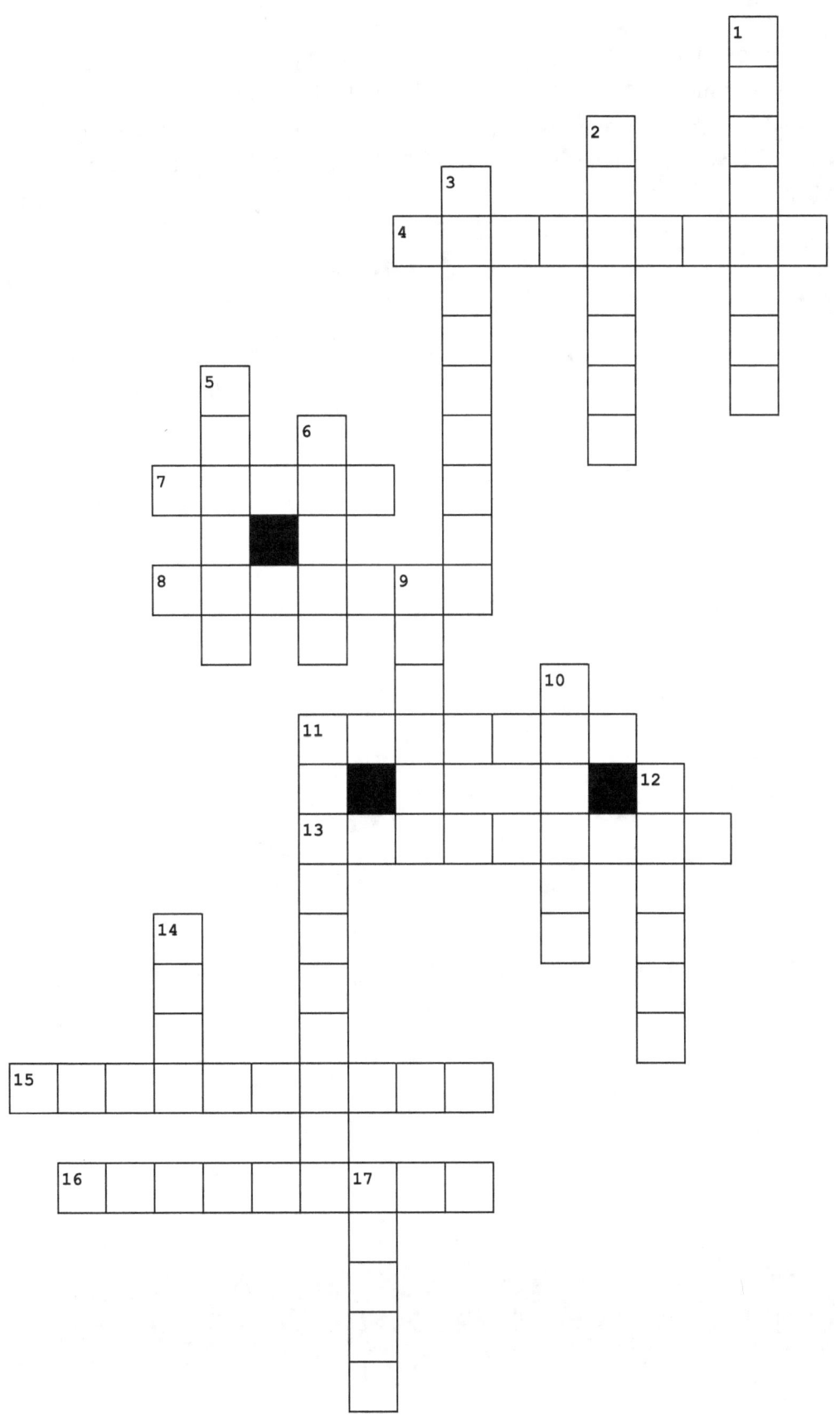

Across

4. ...rhythm
7. ...pressure
8. extreme tiredness
11. desease continuing for a long time
13. when your nose is bleeding
15. a long tube through which food travels while it is being digested after leaving the stomach
16. you have it when you feel dizzy

Down

1. when your head hurts
2. used to hold liquid waste
3. ...processes
5. ...bone
6. to throw up
9. used for carrying a child during pregnancy
10. a medication to stop the pain is a pain...
11. temporary damage to the brain caused by a fall or hit on the head or by violent shaking:
12. ...health
14. to have a runny ...
17. a joint halfway down the arm

NCLEX-26

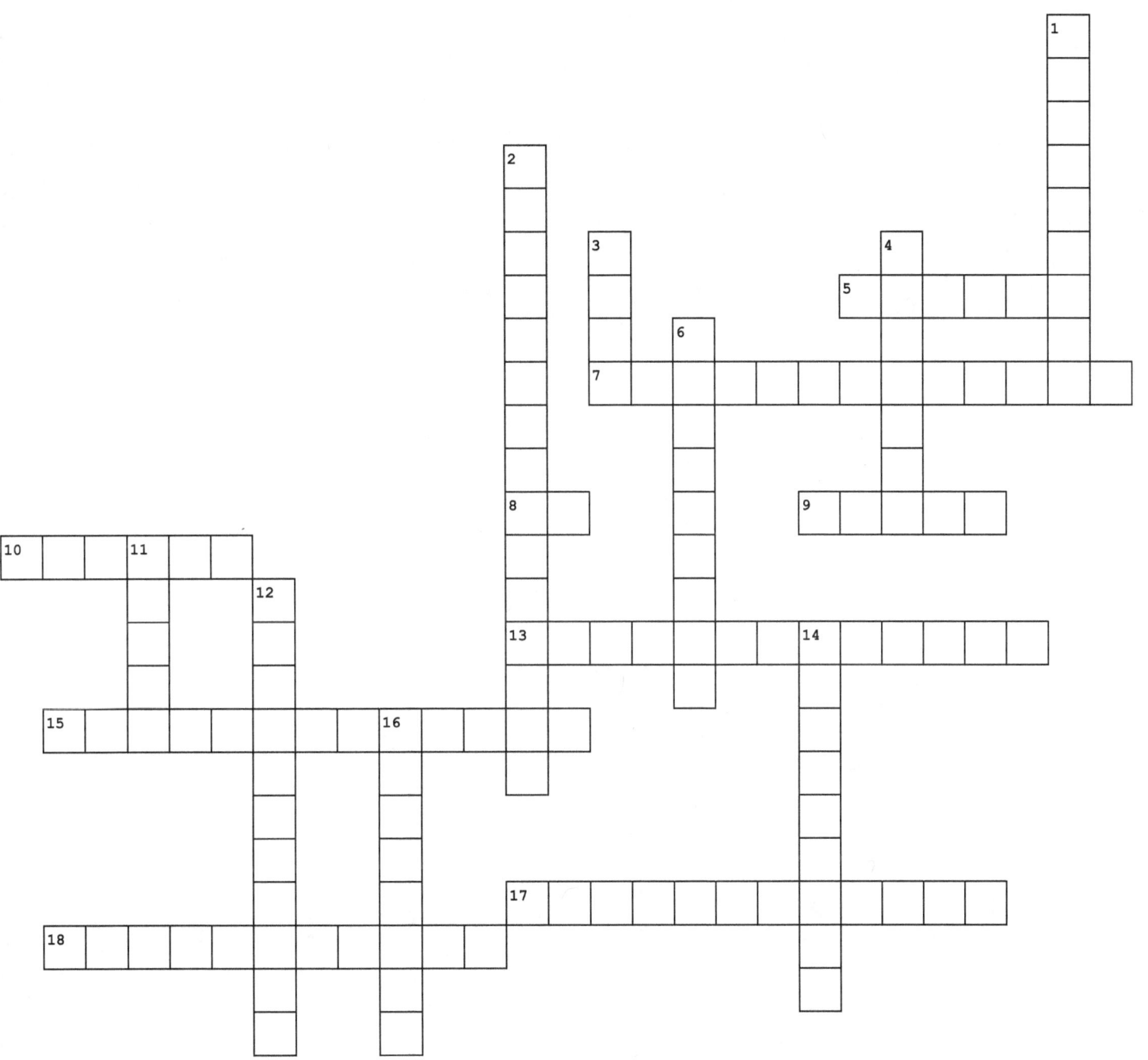

Across
5. used to weigh patient's
7. treats skin conditions
8. where emergency health cases go by Ambulance
9. The number of times your heartbeats
10. An adjustable, wheeled stretcher
13. Treats babies and children
15. Treats blood conditions
17. Treats diseases of the heart

Down
1. Identifying a present disease
2. Helps injured people improve their movement
3. A separate room in a hospital (also called a department)
4. An instrument to cut the skin
6. Predicting the course of a diagnosed illness
11. A qualified health care professional
12. A device used to listen to the heart

18. Used to take a patients temperature

14. A department that performs X-rays

16. A device used to monitor oxygen levels

NCLEX-27

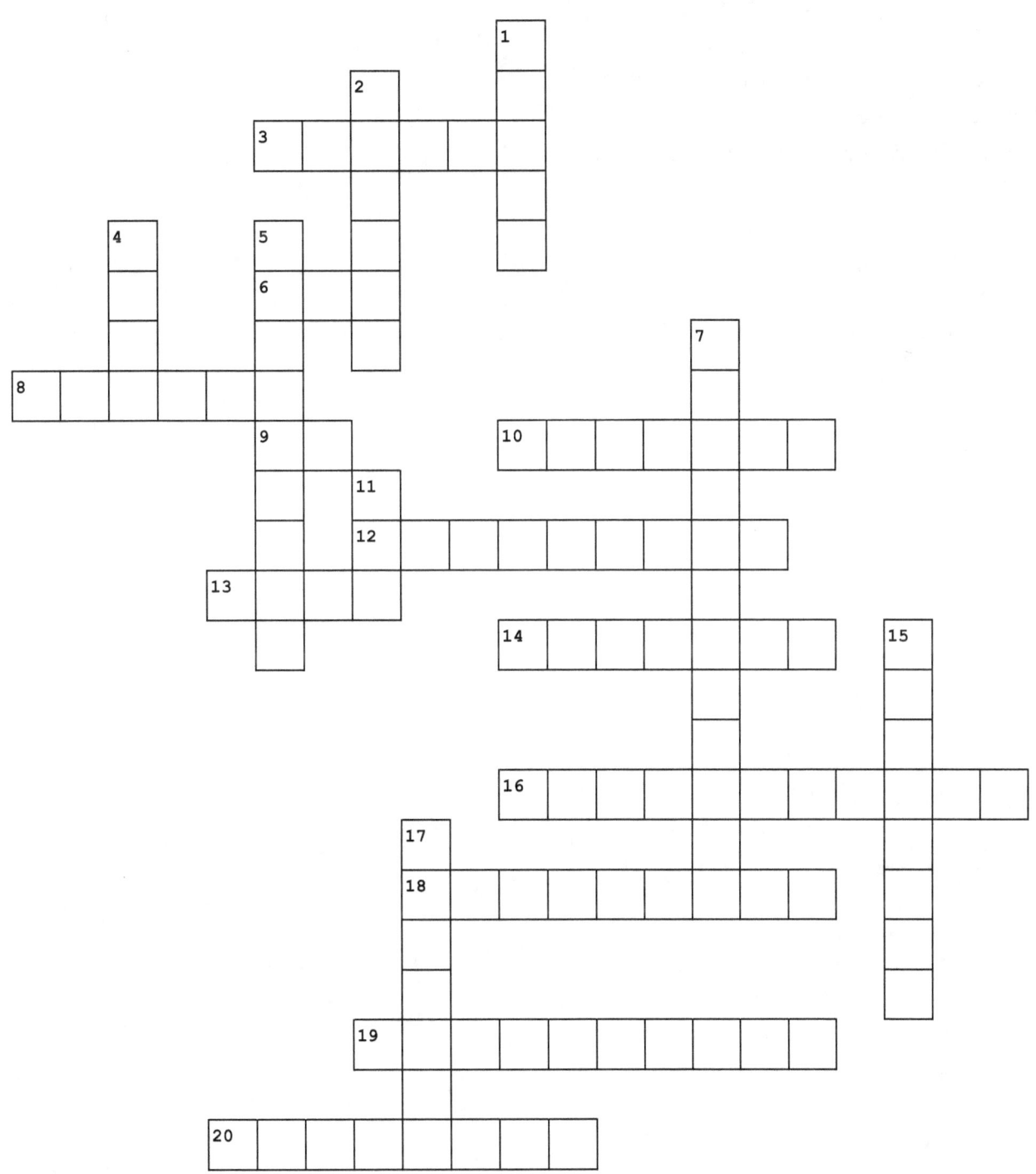

Across

3. - Physician providing medical treatment.
6. - Area for medical testing and analysis.
8. - Essential gas provided to patients in need.
9. - Intravenous, a method of administering fluids or medication.
10. - Medical procedures performed in a hospital.

Down

1. - Medical professional providing patient care.
2. - Uniform worn by medical professionals.
4. - Medical imaging for visualizing internal structures.
5. - Healthcare professional providing direct patient care.

12. - Immediate medical care for urgent situations.
13. - Section of a hospital for a specific type of care.
14. - Preventive treatment to stimulate immunity.
16. - Area for individuals to wait for appointments or news.
18. - Vehicle for transporting patients to the hospital.
19. - Remote healthcare services using technology.
20. - Time for family and friends to see patients in the hospital.

7. - Doctor's written order for medication.
11. - Furniture for patients in a hospital room.
15. - Process of healing and getting better after treatment.
17. - Individual receiving medical treatment.

NCLEX-30

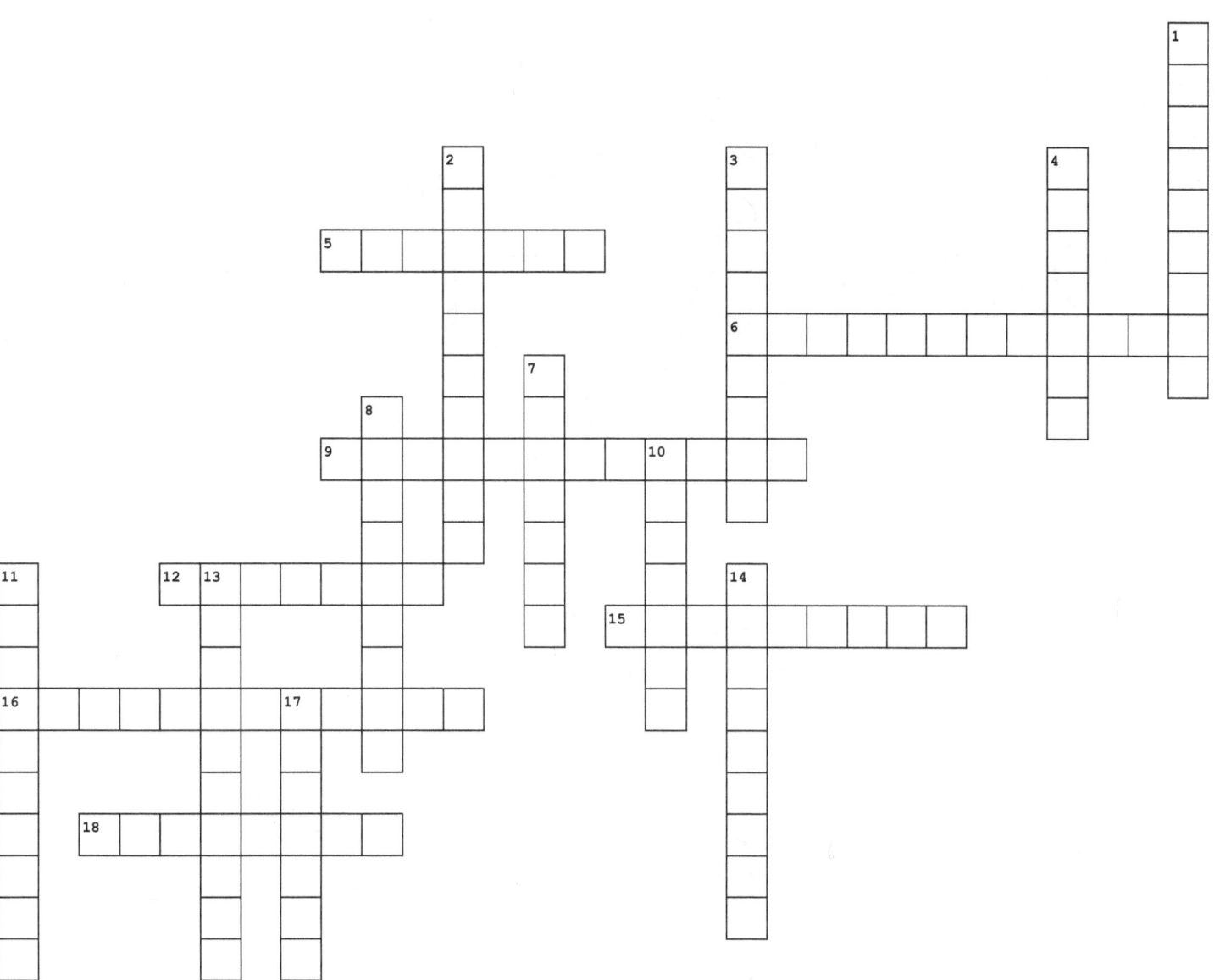

Across
5. A specific abnormal condition affecting the body.
6. A discussion with a healthcare professional.
9. A written order for medication.
12. An individual under medical care.
15. The use of medical imaging technologies.
16. Administration of vaccines to prevent diseases.
18. The period of healing after medical intervention.

Down
1. A plan to manage or cure a medical issue.
2. Loss of sensation during a medical procedure.
3. Invasion of the body by harmful microorganisms.
4. A noticeable change indicating a health issue.
7. Medical procedures involving incisions or manipulation.
8. The expected outcome of a medical condition.
10. Treatments to improve health or well-being.
11. Drugs used to treat medical conditions.
13. A medication to treat bacterial infections.
14. The identification of a disease or condition.
17. An adverse reaction to a specific substance.

NCLEX-16

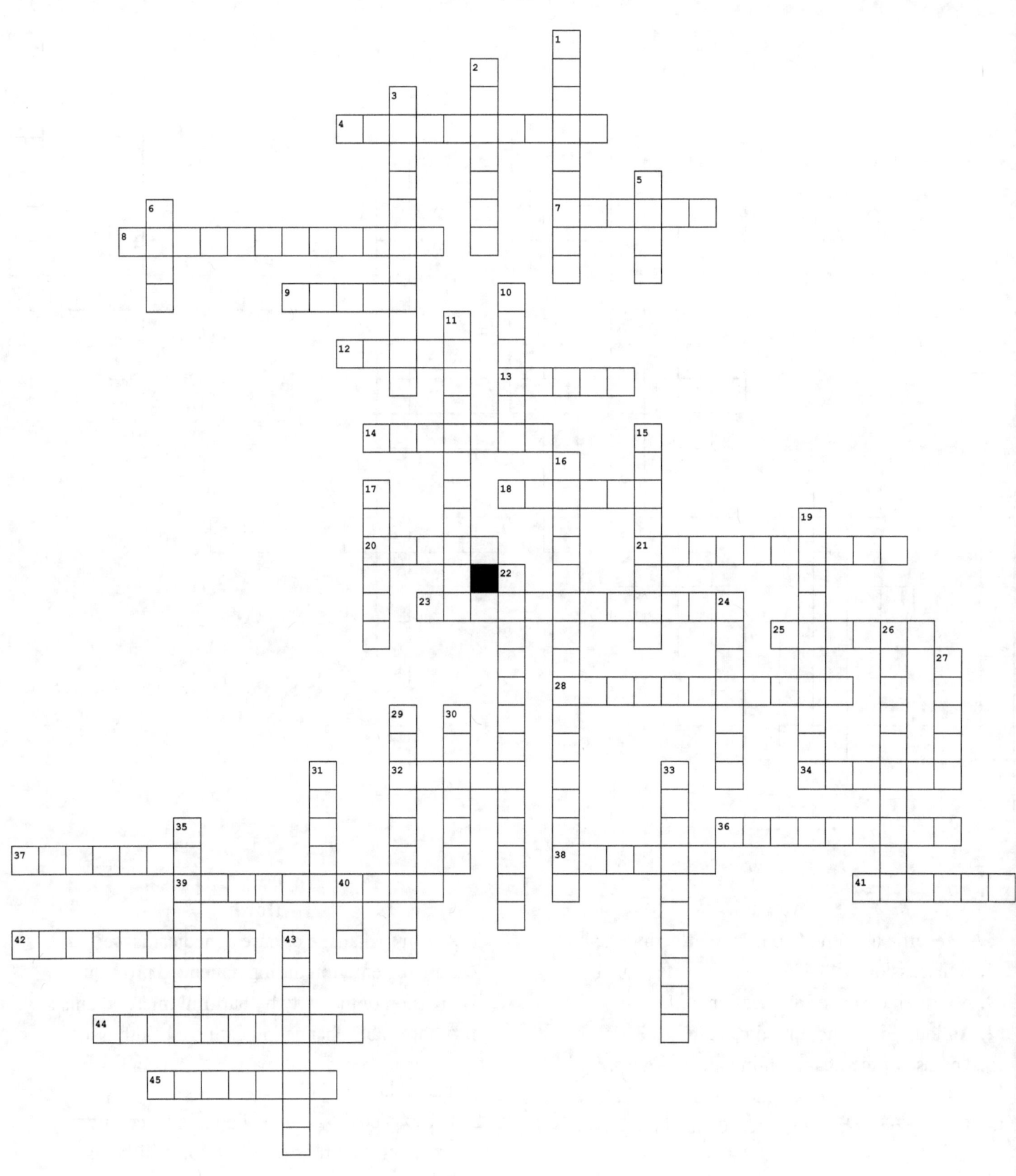

Across

4. a test that examines a urine sample

Down

1. any of the fine branching blood vessels

7. a blood vessel that carries blood away from the heart
8. the use of two or more drugs together to treat a single disease
9. the joint connecting the hand with the forearm
12. the area between the abdomen and the thigh on either side of the body
13. the joint between the forearm and the upper arm
14. the body of contains the digestive organs
18. each of the four slender jointed parts attached to either hand
20. the trunk of the human body
21. a tissue or layer of cells beneath the epidermis
23. the part of the brain that connects the nervous system with the endocrine system
25. a receptacle used by a bedridden patient as a toilet
28. the inability to have children
32. a person trained to care for the sick or infirm
34. breathe out
36. a pain or illness reported by a patient
37. to release by the process of secretion
38. the result of a wrench or twist of the ligaments of a joint
39. any disturbance in the rhythm of the heartbeat
41. an involuntary and immediate movement in response to a stimulus
42. relating to the lungs
44. a chair use as a means of transport by a person who is unable to walk
45. a type of protein found in the body

2. a condition that causes a reaction or illness
3. injury or disability caused when the normal position of a joint
5. a blood vessel that carries blood towards from the heart
6. a protective garment worn in hospital
10. to breathe noisily and with difficulty
11. a procedure to restore blood flow through the artery
15. the part of the face above the eyebrows
16. a doctor who renders the patients unconscious Pharmacist a person who is professionally qualified to prepare and dispense medicinal drugs
17. a respiratory condition, causing difficulty in breathing
19. focusing on preventing diseases from occurring rather than curing them
22. a method of birth control that prevents fertilization of the egg cell
24. a tube with a nozzle and piston for sucking in and ejecting liquid in a thin stream
26. a hormone released into the body of someone feeling extreme emotions
27. a thin translucent fabric of silk, linen, or cotton
29. an injury as from a blow with a blunt instrument
30. a rapid loss of brain functions due to a loss of blood to the brain
31. the part of the human body below the ribs and above the hips
33. the branch of medicine dealing with the diseases and care of aged people
35. a pain felt in the head
40. the sharp edge of a roof from the ridge to the eaves where the two sides meet
43. a waste product found in blood that the kidney usually removes

NCLEX-18

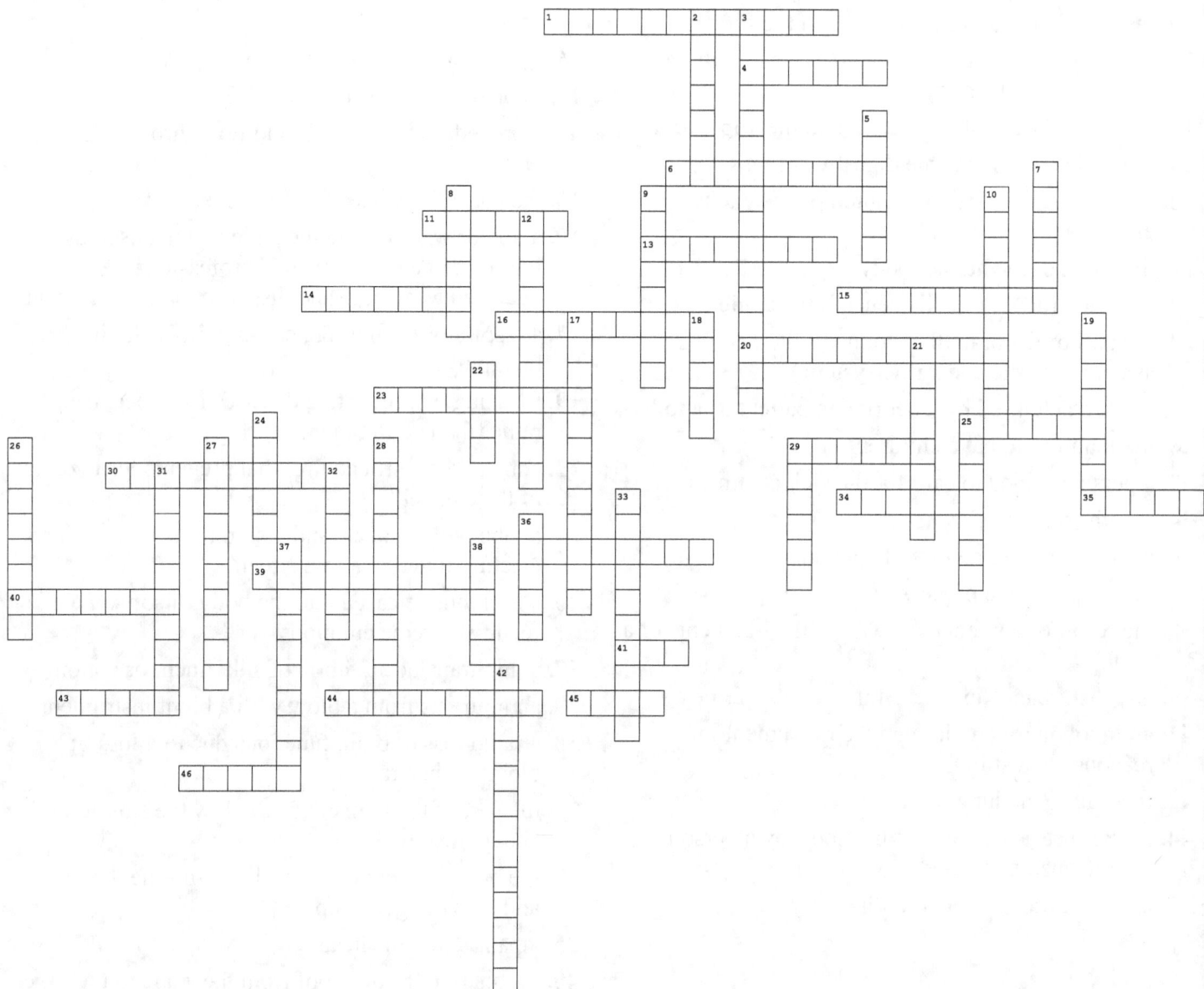

Across

1. the part of the brain that connects the nervous system with the endocrine system
4. breathe out
6. medicine put into a person's body
11. a receptacle used by a bedridden patient as a toilet
13. a hormone that is produced in the ovaries which regulates the menstrual cycle
14. a tube with a nozzle and piston for sucking in and ejecting liquid in a thin stream
15. any of the fine branching blood vessels
16. a pain or illness reported by a patient

Down

2. the body of contains the digestive organs
3. a doctor who renders the patients unconscious
5. each of the four slender jointed parts attached to either hand
7. a blood vessel that carries blood away from the heart
8. an involuntary and immediate movement in response to a stimulus
9. a waste product found in blood that the kidney usually removes
10. a test that examines a urine sample

20. the inability to have children
23. relating to the lungs
25. a respiratory condition, causing difficulty in breathing
29. the result of a wrench or twist of the ligaments of a joint
30. a tissue or layer of cells beneath the epidermis
34. to breathe noisily and with difficulty
35. the joint between the forearm and the upper arm
38. the branch of medicine dealing with the diseases and care of aged people
39. a chair use as a means of transport by a person who is unable to walk
40. a type of protein found in the body
41. the sharp edge of a roof from the ridge to the eaves where the two sides meet
43. a thin translucent fabric of silk, linen, or cotton
44. an injury as from a blow with a blunt instrument
45. a blood vessel that carries blood towards from the heart
46. the part of the human body below the ribs and above the hips

12. a procedure to restore blood flow through the artery
17. the use of two or more drugs together to treat a single disease
18. the trunk of the human body
19. a pain felt in the head
21. having a document saying that a person can do a job
22. a protective garment worn in hospital
24. a person trained to care for the sick or infirm
25. a condition that causes a reaction or illness
26. the part of the face above the eyebrows
27. a hormone released into the body of someone feeling extreme emotions
28. injury or disability caused when the normal position of a joint
29. a rapid loss of brain functions due to a loss of blood to the brain
31. focusing on preventing diseases from occurring rather than curing them
32. to release by the process of secretion
33. any disturbance in the rhythm of the heartbeat
36. the joint connecting the hand with the forearm
37. a person who is professionally qualified to prepare and dispense medicinal drugs
38. the area between the abdomen and the thigh on either side of the body
42. a method of birth control that prevents fertilization of the egg cell

NCLEX-17

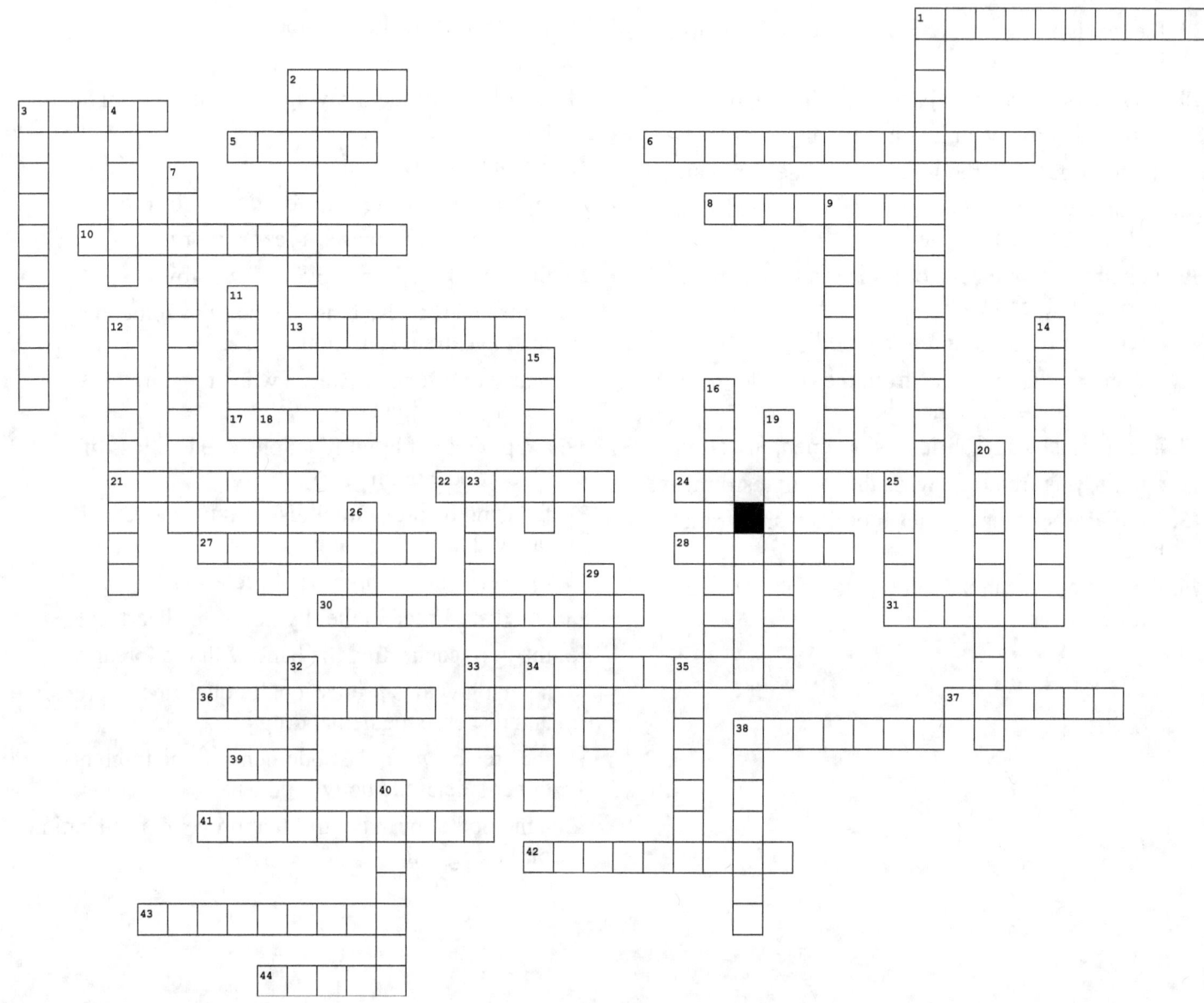

Across

1. a hormone released into the body of someone feeling extreme emotions
2. a protective garment worn in hospital
3. the joint connecting the hand with the forearm
5. the trunk of the human body
6. a method of birth control that prevents fertilization of the egg cell
8. a pain felt in the head
10. injury or disability caused when the normal position of a joint

Down

1. a doctor who renders the patients unconscious
2. the branch of medicine dealing with the diseases and care of aged people
3. a chair use as a means of transport by a person who is unable to walk
4. the result of a wrench or twist of the ligaments of a joint
7. the use of two or more drugs together to treat a single disease
9. any disturbance in the rhythm of the heartbeat
11. the joint between the forearm and the upper arm

13. a waste product found in blood that the kidney usually removes
17. the part of the human body below the ribs and above the hips
21. to release by the process of secretion
22. to breathe noisily and with difficulty
24. a pain or illness reported by a patient
27. the part of the face above the eyebrows
28. an involuntary and immediate movement in response to a stimulus
30. the inability to have children
31. breathe out
33. a procedure to restore blood flow through the artery
36. having a document saying that a person can do a job
37. a respiratory condition, causing difficulty in breathing
38. a type of protein found in the body
39. the sharp edge of a roof from the ridge to the eaves where the two sides meet
41. a test that examines a urine sample
42. relating to the lungs
43. medicine put into a person's
44. a thin translucent fabric of silk, linen, or cotton

12. an injury as from a blow with a blunt instrument
14. focusing on preventing diseases from occurring rather than curing them
15. each of the four slender jointed parts attached to either hand
16. a tissue or layer of cells beneath the epidermis
18. a blood vessel that carries blood away from the heart
19. any of the fine branching blood vessels
20. a person who is professionally qualified to prepare and dispense medicinal drugs
23. the part of the brain that connects the nervous system with the endocrine system
25. a person trained to care for the sick or infirm
26. a blood vessel that carries blood towards from the heart
29. a rapid loss of brain functions due to a loss of blood to the brain
32. a receptacle used by a bedridden patient as a toilet
34. the area between the abdomen and the thigh on either side of the body
35. the body of contains the digestive organs
38. a condition that causes a reaction or illness
40. a tube with a nozzle and piston for sucking in and ejecting liquid in a thin stream

NCLEX-23

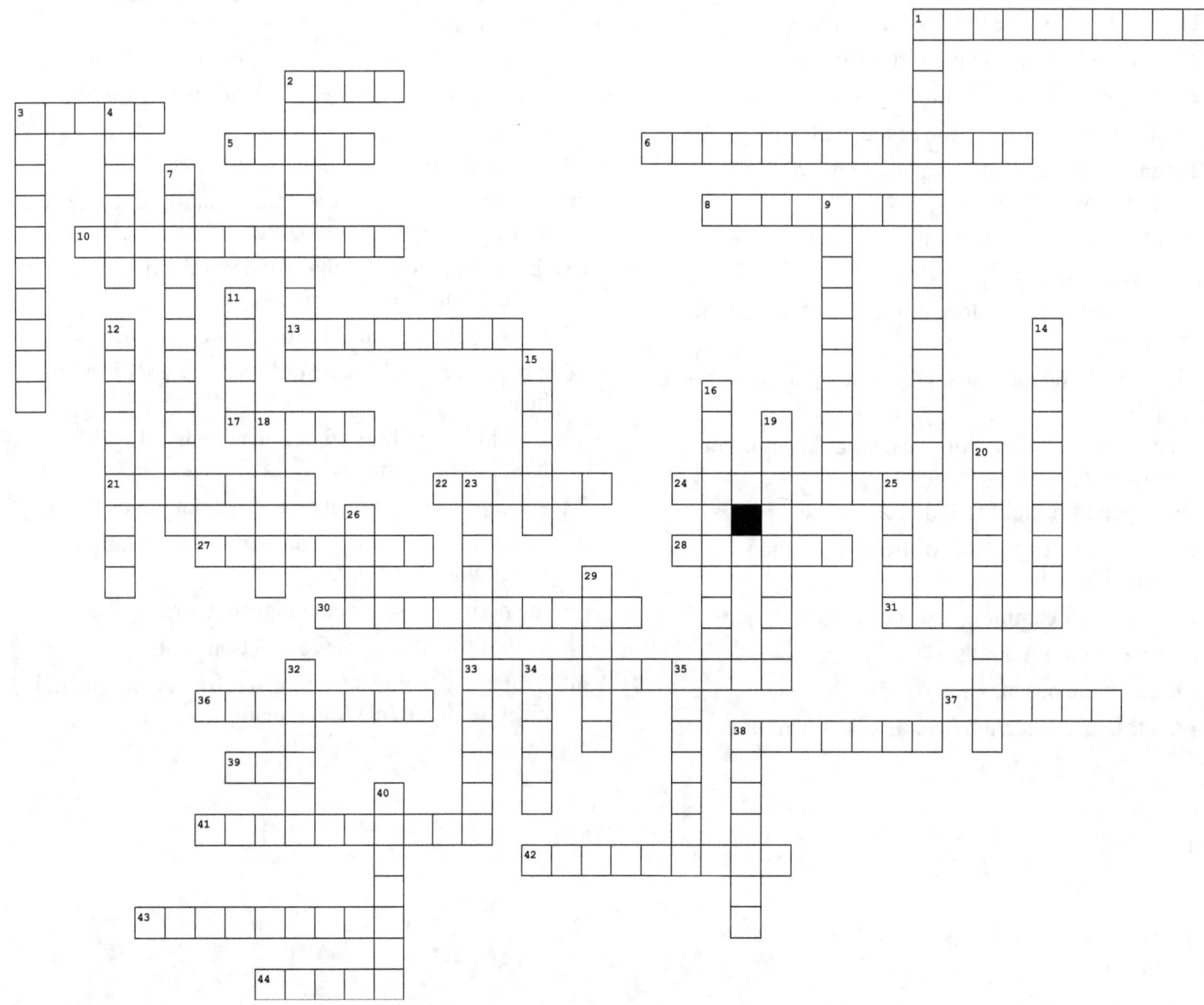

Across

1. a hormone released into the body of someone feeling extreme emotions
2. a protective garment worn in hospital
3. the joint connecting the hand with the forearm
5. the trunk of the human body
6. a method of birth control that prevents fertilization of the egg cell
8. a pain felt in the head
10. injury or disability caused when the normal position of a joint

Down

1. a doctor who renders the patients unconscious
2. the branch of medicine dealing with the diseases and care of aged people
3. a chair use as a means of transport by a person who is unable to walk
4. the result of a wrench or twist of the ligaments of a joint
7. the use of two or more drugs together to treat a single disease
9. any disturbance in the rhythm of the heartbeat
11. the joint between the forearm and the upper arm

13. a waste product found in blood that the kidney usually removes
17. the part of the human body below the ribs and above the hips
21. to release by the process of secretion
22. to breathe noisily and with difficulty
24. a pain or illness reported by a patient
27. the part of the face above the eyebrows
28. an involuntary and immediate movement in response to a stimulus
30. the inability to have children
31. breathe out
33. a procedure to restore blood flow through the artery
36. having a document saying that a person can do a job
37. a respiratory condition, causing difficulty in breathing
38. a type of protein found in the body
39. the sharp edge of a roof from the ridge to the eaves where the two sides meet
41. a test that examines a urine sample
42. relating to the lungs
43. medicine put into a person's
44. a thin translucent fabric of silk, linen, or cotton

12. an injury as from a blow with a blunt instrument
14. focusing on preventing diseases from occurring rather than curing them
15. each of the four slender jointed parts attached to either hand
16. a tissue or layer of cells beneath the epidermis
18. a blood vessel that carries blood away from the heart
19. any of the fine branching blood vessels
20. a person who is professionally qualified to prepare and dispense medicinal drugs
23. the part of the brain that connects the nervous system with the endocrine system
25. a person trained to care for the sick or infirm
26. a blood vessel that carries blood towards from the heart
29. a rapid loss of brain functions due to a loss of blood to the brain
32. a receptacle used by a bedridden patient as a toilet
34. the area between the abdomen and the thigh on either side of the body
35. the body of contains the digestive organs
38. a condition that causes a reaction or illness
40. a tube with a nozzle and piston for sucking in and ejecting liquid in a thin stream

NCLEX-28

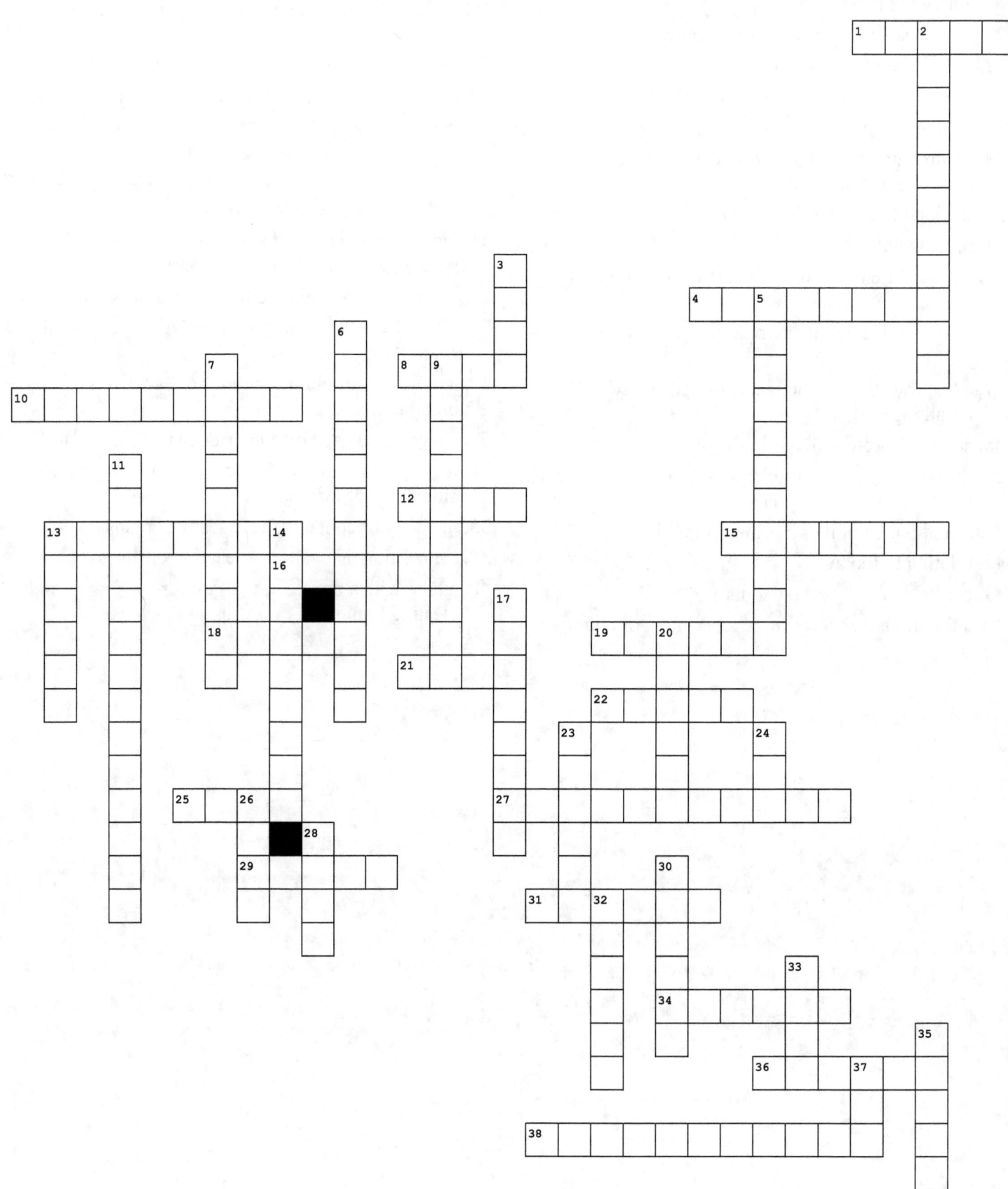

1. Suffix for pain
4. Combining form for vertebrae
8. Prefix for against
10. Medical term for both sides or two sides
12. Prefix for many
13. Combining form for esophagus
15. Suffix for treatment
16. Suffix for paralysis
18. Prefix for within
19. Suffix for surgical repair
21. Suffix for cell
22. Suffix for disease
25. Prefix for below or deficient
27. Medical term for viewing of the joints
29. Suffix for instrument for viewing
31. Suffix for specialist
34. Combining form for liver
36. Suffix for creation of new
38. Medical term for slow heart rate

2. Medical term for surgical removal of stomach
3. Prefix for surrounding or around
5. Medical term for repair of the nose
6. Medical term for enlarged heart
7. Medical term for joint pain
9. Medical term for disease of the nerves
11. Medical term for softening of cartilage
13. Suffix for surgical removal or excision
14. Combining form for eye
17. Medical term for before birth
20. Combining form for joint
23. Combining form for small intestine
24. Combining form for ear
26. Prefix for after or behind
28. Suffix for incision
30. Combining form for mind
32. Combining form for stomach
33. Suffix for inflammation
35. Prefix above or excessive
37. Suffix for tumor

NCLEX-29

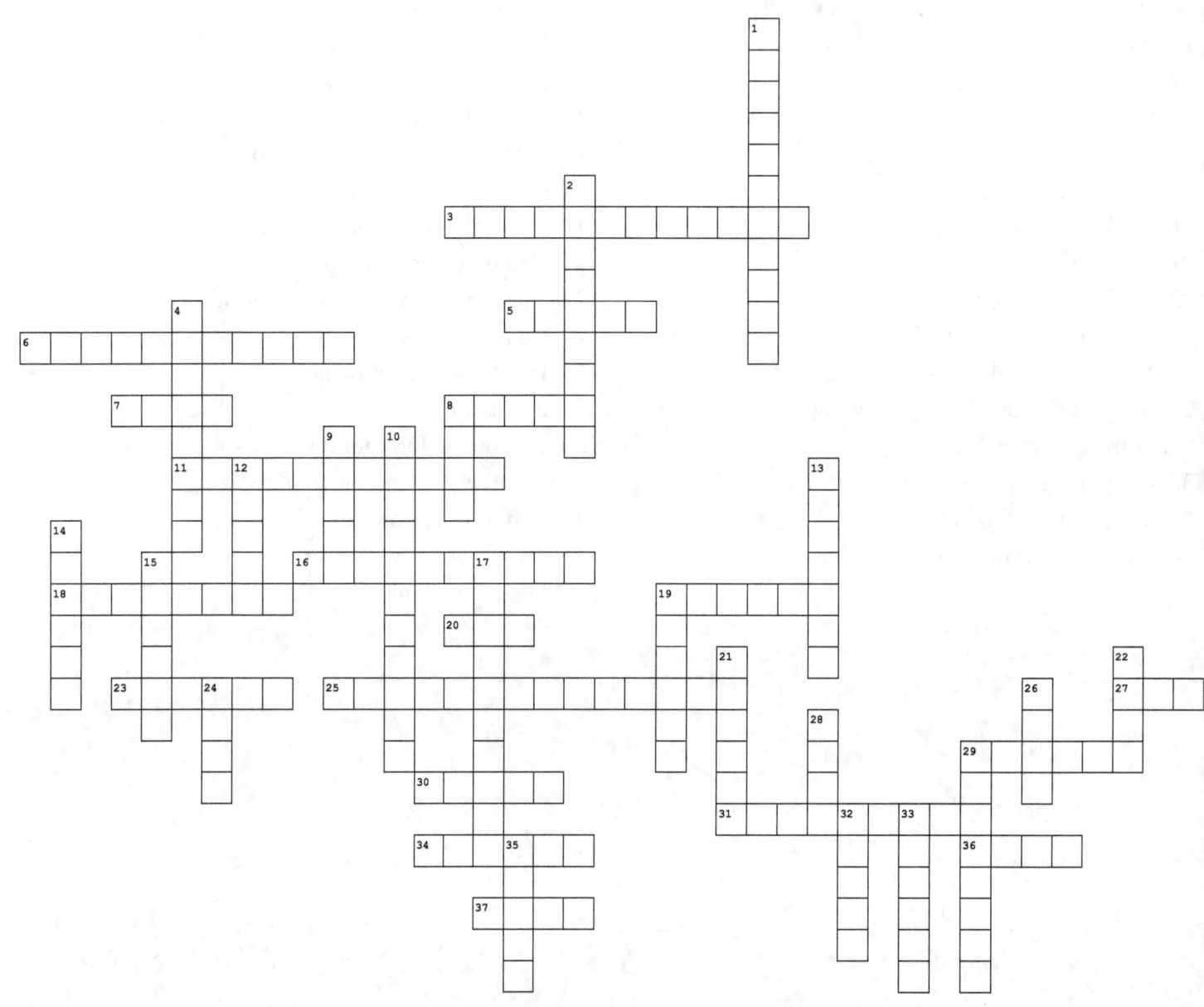

Across
3. Medical term for enlarged heart
5. Suffix for Disease
6. Medical term for removal of stomach
7. Prefix for against
8. Suffix for in or within
11. Medical Term for Slow Heart Rate
16. Medical term for disease of the nerves
18. Medical Term for before birth
19. Suffix for paralysis
20. Combining form for Ear
23. Combining form for Joint

Down
1. Surgical repair of the nose
2. Medical Term for both (two) sides
4. Combining form for Vertebrae
8. Suffix for inflammation
9. Suffix for instrument for viewing
10. Medical Term for viewing the Joints
12. Suffix for pain
13. Suffix for Treatment
14. Combining form for Liver
15. Combining form for small intestine
17. Medical term for joint pain

25. Medical term for softening of the cartilage
27. Suffix for tumor
29. Medical term for surgical removal;excision
30. Suffix for pain
31. Combining form for Eye
34. Suffix for surgical repair
36. Prefix for around or surrounding
37. Prefix for Many

19. Combining form for Mind
21. Combining form for stomach
22. Suffix for incision
24. Suffix for below or deficient
26. Suffix for Cell
28. Prefix for after or behind
29. Combining form for Esophagus
32. prefix for above or excessive
33. Suffix for specialist
35. Suffix for Surgical opening

Answers:

NCLEX-1:
across • aden • arm • bone • breathing • chest • cyan • cyte • dent • ectomy • edema • endo • exo • heart • hyper •
hypo • itis • lung • nas • nerve • pulse • red • rib • scler • skin • stomach • sugar • thromb

NCLEX-2:
appendix • arthr • asthenia • blast • edema • gravid • iris • itis • lept • maxill • ovario • phage • phob • phon • phot •
plexus • rrhe • tarso • thalam • ton

NCLEX-3:
air • dist • divided • grape • kenesis • love • lumb • man • meta • month • nucleus • pan • paralysis • pus • squam •
tachy • tarso • tome • upward • vivi

NCLEX-4:
adrenalo • amigo • c/o • centesis • chest • dys- • ectomy • head • hemato • hyper • irony- • joint • kidney • lukeo- •
malaria • neo- • osis • ostomy- • peri- • rrhea • rrhexis • scope • stomach • uterus • yacht-

NCLEX-5:
ANOREXIA • Anxiety • ARTERIOCLEROSIS • Behaviorism • bone • breathe • BULIMIA • CHEST • DETENTION • Development • ECTOMY • EDEMA • HEART • Hemoglobin • HYPO • INFECTION • Manic • Psychology • PULSE • Resilience • RIB • SKIN • SMALL • STOMACH • Stress

NCLEX-6:
ANOREXIA • Anxiety • ARTERIOCLEROSIS • Behaviorism • bone • breathe • BULIMIA • CHEST • DETENTION • Development • ECTOMY • EDEMA • HEART • Hemoglobin • HYPO • INFECTION • Manic • Psychology • PULSE • Resilience • RIB • SKIN • SMALL • STOMACH • Stress

NCLEX-7:
ANOREXIA • Anxiety • ARTERIOCLEROSIS • Behaviorism • bone • breathe • BULIMIA • CHEST • DETENTION • Development • ECTOMY • EDEMA • HEART • Hemoglobin • HYPO • INFECTION • Manic • Psychology • PULSE • Resilience • RIB • SKIN • SMALL • STOMACH • Stress • Superego

NCLEX-8:
Anorexia,Medical • Cardiologist, • Dehydration, • Dermatologist, • Diabetes, • Epilepsy, • Hemoglobin, •
Hypertension, • Hypoglycemia, • Hypokalemia, • Insomnia, • Leukocytes, • Lyme, • Malaria, • Melatonin, •
Mumps, • Polyuria, • Rabies, • Renal, • Rubella, • Scurvy, • Tachycardia • Tachypnea, • Thyroid

NCLEX-9:
anesthesiologist • bedpan • bone • cardiology • department • dermatology • emergency • gauze • gown • joint • nurse • obstetrics • orthopedics • oxygen • pathology • pediatrics • pharmacy • practitioner • pregnancy • prescription • procedure • radiology • sample • surgery • syringe • technician • threatening • treatment • wheelchair

NCLEX-10:
abduct • adduct • anesthetist • cardiologist • cyan • dementia • dermatology • dietary • digits • gynecology • melan • micro • optician • orthopedics • patella • pediatrics • podiartist • posterior • psychiatry • respiratory • surgical • toxoid • urinary • venous

NCLEX-11:
analgesics • anorexics • antacids • antibiotics • anticoagulants • anticonvulsants • antidepressants • antiemetics • antihistamines • antipyretics • antitussives • bronchodilators • cathartics • diuretics • dog • heartdepressants • hormones • ironcompounds • musculoskeletalrelaxants • respiratorystimulants • sedatives • tranquilizers • vitamins

NCLEX-12:
analgesics • anorexics • antacids • antibiotics • anticoagulants • anticonvulsants • antidepressants • antiemetics •antihistamines • antipyretics • antitussives • bronchodilators • cathartics • diuretics • dog • heartdepressants •

hormones • ironcompounds • musculoskeletalrelaxants • respiratorystimulants • sedatives • tranquilizers • vitamins

NCLEX-13:
brainstem • bronchi • copd • cough • diaphragm • diastolicblood • dorsalispedispulse • exercise • ild • image • intercostalmusclestrain • kinesiology • moderna • myocardialinfarction • oxygen • pleurisy • pneumonia • pulmonary • pulserate • right • sixhundred • tad • thirtysix • thoraciccage • trachea • two • twohundredsix

NCLEX-14:
Ante • Bilateral • Blepharo • Cardio • Cherry • Comedo • Dysmenorrhea • Encephalo • Endo • Erythrocyte • Eupepsia • Hepato • Hirutism • Incontinence • Menarche • Myocardial • Nephro • Oophorocytosis • Osteoporosis • Phrenospasm • Pulmono • Somnambulism • Spleno • Spondylo • Superior • Tinnitus

NCLEX-15:
amniocentesis • asystole • bromodosis • cardiomegaly • cholecystectomy • colonoscopy • computedtomography • diabeticketoacidosis • fracture • hyoid • hyster • keloid • leukocyte • npo • occipital • patella • potassium • pots • radiationtherapy • transientischemicattack • trisomy

NCLEX-16:
abdomen • adrenaline • albumin • allergy • anesthesiologist • angioplasty • arrhythmia • artery • asthma • bedpan • capillary • complaint • contraceptive • contusion • creatine • dislocation • elbow • exhale • finger • forehead • gauze • geriatrics • gown • groin • headache • hip • hypodermis • hypothalamus • infertility • nurse • polypharmacy • preventive • pulmonary • reflex • secrete • sprain • stroke • syringe • torso • urinalysis • vein • waist • wheelchair • wheeze • wrist

NCLEX-17:
abdomen • adrenaline • albumin • allergy • anesthesiologist • angioplasty • arrhythmia • artery • asthma • bedpan • capillary • complaint • contraceptive • contusion • creatine • dislocation • elbow • exhale • finger • forehead • gauze • geriatrics • gown • groin • headache • hip • hypodermis • hypothalamus • infertility • injection • licensed • nurse • pharmacist • polypharmacy • preventive • pulmonary • reflex • secrete • sprain • stroke • syringe • torso • urinalysis • vein • waist • wheelchair • wheeze • wrist

NCLEX-18:
abdomen • adrenaline • albumin • allergy • anesthesiologist • angioplasty • arrhythmia • artery • asthma • bedpan • capillary • complaint • contraceptive • contusion • creatine • dislocation • elbow • estrogen • exhale • finger • forehead • gauze • geriatrics • gown • groin • headache • hip • hypodermis • hypothalamus • infertility • injection • licensed • nurse • pharmacist • polypharmacy • preventive • pulmonary • reflex • secrete • sprain • stroke • syringe • torso • urinalysis • vein • waist • wheelchair • wheeze • wrist

NCLEX-19:
aurus • branchium • cerebrum • cor • corpus • crus • dens • digitus • frons • iuglem • labium • linga • manus • nas • oculus • pes • sangis • umerus • vena • venter

NCLEX-20:

aneurysm • apex • base • bld • bp • bpm • cardi(o) • coronary • cv • echo • echocardiogram • electrocardiogram • endocardium • epicardium • hem(o) • hypertension • interatrial • myocardial • myocardium • sphygmomanometer • thoracic • varicose

NCLEX-21:
analgesics • anorexics • antacids • antibiotics • anticoagulants • anticonvulsants • antidepressants • antiemetics • antihistamines • antipyretics • antitussives • bronchodilators • cathartics • diuretics • dog • heartdepressants • hormones • ironcompounds • musculoskeletalrelaxants • respiratorystimulants • sedatives • tranquilizers • vitamins

NCLEX-22:
blood • cough • decease • diagnosis • drugs • fever • injection • medicine • nurse • pharmacy • plaster • prescribe • proper • scar • surgery • symptom • temperature • treat • vaccination • wound

NCLEX-23:
abdomen • adrenaline • albumin • allergy • anesthesiologist • angioplasty • arrhythmia • artery • asthma • bedpan • capillary • complaint • contraceptive • contusion • creatine • dislocation • elbow • exhale • finger • forehead • gauze • geriatrics • gown • groin • headache • hip • hypodermis • hypothalamus • infertility • injection • licensed • nurse • pharmacist • polypharmacy • preventive • pulmonary • reflex • secrete • sprain • stroke • syringe • torso • urinalysis • vein • waist • wheelchair • wheeze • wrist

NCLEX-24:
Dermatologist • Diagnosis • Electrocardiogram • ER • Gurney • Haematologist • Nurse • Oximeter • Paediatrician • Physiotherapist • Prognosis • Pulse • Radiology • Scales • Scalpel • Stethoscope • Thermometer • Treats • Ward

NCLEX-25:
bladder • blood • chronic • circadian • collar • concussion • digestive • dizziness • elbow • fatigue • headache • intestines • killer • mental • nose • nosebleed • uterus • vomit

NCLEX-26:
Cardiologist • Dermatologist • Diagnosis • Er • Gurney • Haematologist • Nurse • Oximetry • Paediatrician • Physiotherapist • Prognosis • Pulse • Radiology • Scales • Scalpel • Stethoscope • Thermometer • Ward

NCLEX-27:
AMBULANCE • BED • CLINICIAN • DOCTOR • EMERGENCY • IV • LAB • NURSE • OXYGEN • PATIENT • PRESCRIPTION • RECOVERY • SCRUBS • SURGERY • TELEHEALTH • VACCINE • VISITING • WAITINGROOM • WARD • XRAY

NCLEX-28:

algia • anti • arthralgia • arthro • arthroscopy • bilateral • bradycardia • cardiomegaly • chondromalacia • cyte • ectomy • entero • esophago • gastrectomy • gastro • hepato • hyper • hypo • iatrics • intra • itis • logist • neuropathy • oma • ophthalmo • ostomy • oto • pathy • peri • plasty • plegia • poly • post • prenatal • psycho • rhinoplasty • scope • tomy • vertebro

NCLEX-29:

algia • algia • anti • arthralgia • arthro • arthroscopy • bilateral • bradycardia • cardiomegaly • chondromalacia • cyte • ectomy • entero • esophago • gastrectomy • gastro • hepato • hyper • hypo • intra • itis • logist • neuropathy • oma • ophthalmo • oto • pathy • peri • plasty • plegia • poly • post • prenatal • psycho • rhinoplasty • scope • stomy • therapy • tomy • vertebro

NCLEX-30:

Allergy • Anesthesia • Antibiotic • Consultation • Diagnosis • Disease • Immunization • Infection • Medication • Patient • Prescription • Prognosis • Radiology • Recovery • Surgery • Symptom • Therapy • Treatment

www.ingramcontent.com/pod-product-compliance
Lightning Source LLC
Chambersburg PA
CBHW062123220526
45471CB00010B/3861